A Doctor's Practical Guide to Understanding & Managing

GALL BLADDER STONES & OTHER DISEASES

Dr Prabhat Das

MD, PhD, FACP

Better Health with Dr Das Series

Hardcover ISBN: 978-1-971672-33-5

Paperback ISBN: 978-1-971672-32-8

eBook ISBN: 978-1-971672-31-1

Printed in the United States of America

Disclaimer

This book is intended solely for educational and informational purposes. It is not meant to replace personal medical advice, diagnosis, or treatment.

Although I am a licensed physician, reading this book does not establish a doctor-patient relationship. Each individual's health condition, medical history, and risk factors are unique. Any medical decision should be made in partnership with your own healthcare professional who understands your specific situation.

Medical science is continually advancing. New research and updated guidelines may lead to changes in recommendations over time.

TABLE OF CONTENTS:

About the Author

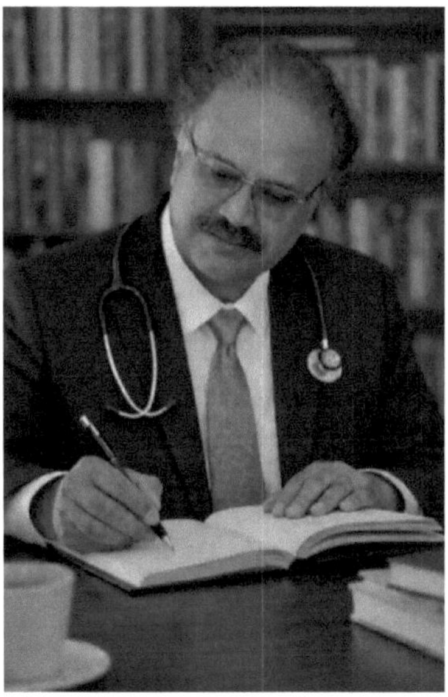

I am Dr Prabhat Das, MD, PhD, FACP. My journey in medicine began in India and, over the past thirty-five years, has continued in the United States, where I have had the privilege of caring for patients across a wide range of medical settings. I am trained in Internal Medicine,

Pulmonary Diseases, and Critical Care. For me, medicine has never been just a profession. It has been a lifelong commitment shaped by learning, service, and a deep respect for the trust patients place in their physician.

Over the years, I have had the honor of caring for patients in many different situations. I have seen individuals in my office for routine concerns, treated urgent conditions in busy emergency rooms, managed serious illnesses in the hospital, and cared for critically ill patients in intensive care units. Each setting has taught me something valuable. Each patient has added to my understanding of what it truly means to care for another human being.

But one lesson has stood above all others. Medicine is not only about tests, diagnoses, or treatments. It is about people. It is about listening carefully, understanding fears that are often left unspoken, and guiding patients through uncertainty with clarity and compassion. Again and again, I have seen that what people want most is simple, trustworthy information. They want to understand what is happening in their bodies. They want to feel confident about the decisions they are making for their health and for their families.

These experiences have deeply shaped how I think about health, illness, prevention, and the human side of healing.

That is the reason behind the '**Better Health with Dr Das Series**'. Through these books, I hope to reach individuals I may never meet in person but who are searching for clear and reliable guidance. In today's world, health information is everywhere, yet much of it is confusing, overwhelming, and sometimes misleading. My goal is to cut through that noise and present important medical topics in a way that is simple, practical, and reassuring.

Every page of this series is guided by two foundations: reliable scientific knowledge and decades of real-world clinical experience. I want you, the reader, to feel informed, confident, and empowered. Not overwhelmed. Not confused. But clear about what you can do, step by step, to improve your health.

If even one reader feels less anxious, more informed, or better prepared to take control of their health after reading these books, then this work has served its purpose.

Helping people live healthier, longer, more confident and better-informed lives remains one of the greatest privileges of my life.

CHAPTER 1: Why Gallbladder Health Matters More Than Most People Realize

A Small Organ Most People Never Think About

Most people go through life without ever thinking about their gallbladder. It quietly does its job in the background, and as long as everything is working well, there is no reason to notice it.

That changes the moment something goes wrong.

The gallbladder is a small, pear-shaped organ tucked under the liver on the right side of the abdomen. Its role is simple but important. It stores and releases bile, a fluid that helps digest fats. When this process works smoothly, digestion feels effortless. When it does not, even a simple meal can become uncomfortable.

Over the years, I have seen this pattern again and again. A person who never had digestive issues suddenly begins to feel pain after meals, a sense of heaviness, nausea, or bloating. At first, it is dismissed as gas or acidity. Then the episodes return. Eventually, one attack becomes severe enough to bring the person to medical attention.

That is when the gallbladder finally comes into focus.

A Common Problem That Is Often Overlooked

Gallbladder disease is far more common than most people realize. Gallstones, in particular, are among the most frequent digestive conditions seen in medical practice.

Many people have gallstones and never know it. These are called silent stones. They cause no symptoms and may never need treatment.

But in some individuals, the story is very different.

Stones begin to interfere with the normal flow of bile. Pain starts to appear, often after meals. Episodes may be mild at first, then gradually become more frequent or intense. In some cases, complications such as inflammation, infection, or blockage of the bile ducts can develop.

What makes this condition important is this wide range. It can be completely silent in one person and significantly disruptive in another.

Why Early Symptoms Are Often Missed

One of the reasons gallbladder disease is often delayed in diagnosis is the nature of early symptoms.

They are usually not dramatic.

A person may feel:

A vague discomfort in the upper abdomen

A sense of fullness after eating

Mild nausea

Occasional bloating

These symptoms are easy to ignore. Most people attribute them to overeating, stress, or something they ate.

And sometimes, the discomfort does pass.

But then it returns.

This pattern is important. Recurrent symptoms, even if mild, are often the body's way of signaling that something is not quite right.

Why Understanding This Condition Matters

A good health book should do more than define medical terms. It should help you make sense of what your body is telling you and guide you toward the right decisions.

That is the purpose of this book.

Here, I will walk you through:

How the gallbladder works

How gallstones form

Why some people develop symptoms while others do not

How to recognize early warning signs

When to seek medical care

What tests are used and why

When surgery is needed and what it involves

What to expect after treatment

How diet and lifestyle affect long-term health

Everything will be explained in clear, simple language, without losing accuracy.

Clearing Confusion and Misinformation

Gallbladder disease is surrounded by a surprising amount of confusion.

Some people are told that all gallstones must be removed. Others are told that surgery should always be avoided. Many hear about quick remedies that promise to dissolve stones naturally.

These mixed messages create uncertainty.

The truth lies somewhere in between.

Some gallstones never cause problems and do not require treatment. Others, once symptomatic, are best managed with a definitive approach. Diet plays a role, but it cannot remove existing stones. And while some treatments may help in selected cases, there is no universal shortcut.

Reliable, balanced information is essential to make the right decision.

More Than Just Gallstones

Although gallstones are the most common issue, the gallbladder can be affected in other ways as well.

These include:

Inflammation of the gallbladder

Blockage of bile ducts

Functional problems where the gallbladder does not empty properly

Sludge and microscopic stones

Polyps and structural changes

Rarely, more serious conditions

Understanding this broader picture helps you avoid oversimplifying the problem.

The Real Goal of This Book

My goal is not to create fear.

It is to replace confusion with clarity.

By the time you finish this book, you should feel:

More confident in understanding your symptoms

More comfortable discussing your condition with your doctor

Better prepared to make decisions about treatment

More in control of your health

When you understand what is happening inside your body, everything becomes easier.

A Thought from My Practice

Over the years, I have learned a simple truth.

Most gallbladder problems can be managed effectively when they are understood early and handled appropriately. The difficulty usually arises when symptoms are ignored, misunderstood, or delayed.

Awareness makes a difference.

Chapter Summary

The gallbladder is a small but important organ involved in digestion. Gallbladder disease, especially gallstones, is common and may be silent or symptomatic. Early symptoms are often mild and overlooked, but recurring patterns should not be ignored.

Action Plan

Pay attention to your body, especially after meals. If you notice recurring discomfort, nausea, or bloating, do not dismiss it repeatedly as simple indigestion. If you have already been diagnosed with gallstones, begin observing whether symptoms are present and how often they occur.

Transition to Next Chapter

Now that we have set the foundation, the next step is to understand how the gallbladder and the entire bile system actually work.

CHAPTER 2: Understanding the Gallbladder, Bile, and the Biliary System

Building a Clear Mental Picture

Before we go further, pause for a moment and form a simple picture in your mind.

In my experience, once patients understand how this system works under normal conditions, everything else becomes easier. Symptoms make sense. Test results feel less confusing. Treatment decisions feel more logical.

You do not need complex anatomy. You need a clear, practical understanding.

Where the Gallbladder Is Located

The gallbladder sits just beneath the liver on the right side of the upper abdomen.

It is small and usually not felt under normal conditions. It remains quietly tucked under the liver, doing its job without drawing attention.

Because it lies close to the stomach, liver, and pancreas, problems in this area can sometimes feel similar. This is one reason symptoms can be confusing.

The Liver – The Source of Bile

The liver is the main organ in this system.

It produces bile continuously, whether you are eating or not.

Bile contains:

Bile salts that help digest fats

Cholesterol

Bilirubin, a waste product

Water and other substances

This balance is important. When it changes, especially with excess cholesterol, stones can begin to form.

The Gallbladder – Storage and Timing

The gallbladder does not produce bile. Its role is to store and concentrate it.

Between meals:

Bile flows from the liver into the gallbladder

It is stored and becomes concentrated

When you eat, especially fatty food:

The gallbladder contracts

Bile is released into the intestine

This timing helps digestion work smoothly.

The Bile Ducts – The Pathway

Bile travels through a network of ducts.

A simple way to understand the flow:

The liver produces bile

Small ducts carry it outward

These join to form larger ducts

The gallbladder connects through the cystic duct

The common bile duct carries bile to the intestine

This pathway is essential. If it is blocked, problems begin.

What Happens When You Eat

Let us follow the process step by step.

When you eat, especially fatty food:

Signals are sent to the gallbladder

The gallbladder contracts

Bile is released into the intestine

Bile helps break down fats for absorption

When everything works well, you are not aware of it.

When the System Is Disturbed

Problems arise when this flow is interrupted.

This can happen when:

Stones form

The gallbladder does not empty properly

A stone blocks the duct

The result may be:

Pain

Inflammation

Infection

Jaundice

This is why understanding bile flow is so important.

The Link with the Pancreas

There is one important connection.

The bile duct joins the pancreatic duct before entering the intestine.

Because of this:

A blockage can affect both systems

This explains gallstone pancreatitis

This connection is clinically important.

A Simple Way to Remember

If you remember just three points, you will understand most of this system:

The liver makes bile

The gallbladder stores and releases bile

The ducts carry bile to the intestine

When any part is blocked or not functioning well, symptoms develop.

Why This Understanding Matters

This is not just theory.

When you understand this system:

Pain patterns make sense

Symptoms feel less confusing

Test reports become clearer

Treatment decisions feel logical

This knowledge builds confidence.

A Thought from My Practice

I have often noticed that once patients understand this simple flow, their anxiety reduces significantly. The unknown becomes familiar, and that makes a real difference.

Gallbladder System

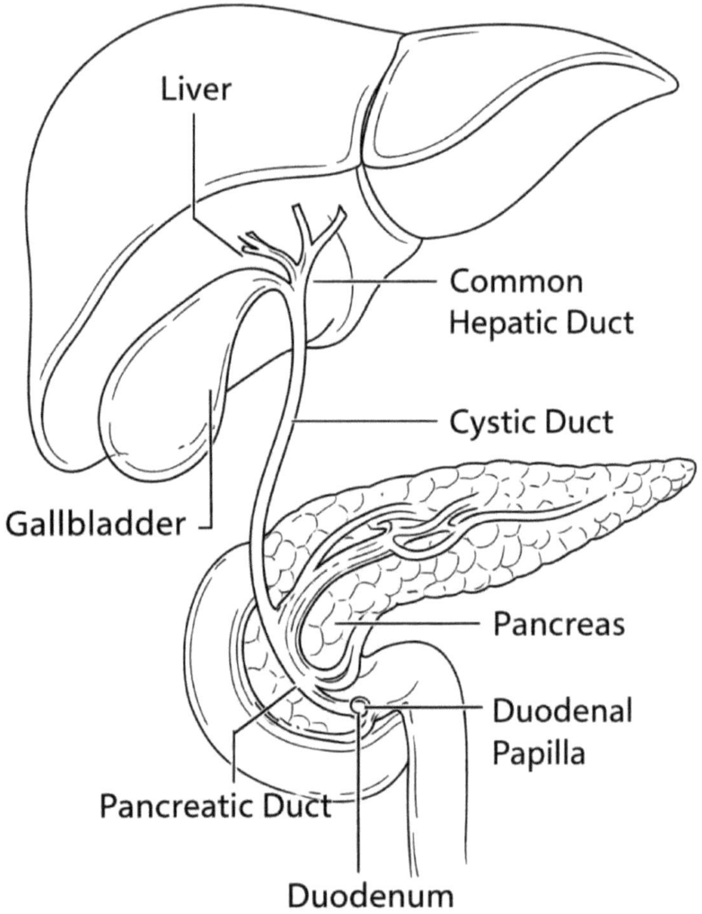

Chapter Summary

The gallbladder stores bile produced by the liver. Bile helps digest fats and flows through a system of ducts into the intestine. Problems occur when this flow is disrupted by stones, poor emptying, or blockage.

Action Plan

Begin observing how your body responds to meals, especially fatty meals. If symptoms occur, note their timing and pattern. This simple awareness will help you and your doctor greatly.

Transition to Next Chapter

Now that you understand how the system works, the next step is to see what can go wrong within it and how different gallbladder conditions are connected.

CHAPTER 3: The Big Picture – What Can Go Wrong in the Gallbladder

Seeing the Whole Landscape First

Before we go deeper into individual conditions, it helps to step back and look at the entire picture.

In my experience, many patients focus only on one term, usually "gallstones," and assume that is the whole story. But gallbladder disease is broader. Stones are often the starting point, but they can lead to several different problems.

When you understand the full landscape, you stop feeling lost. You begin to see where your own situation fits.

Gallstones – The Most Common Starting Point

The most frequent problem is the formation of gallstones.

These are solid deposits that develop when bile loses its normal balance. In many people, stones remain silent and never cause symptoms. In others, they begin to cause trouble.

According to the National Institute of Diabetes and Digestive and Kidney Diseases, gallstones are common and often discovered incidentally, but symptomatic stones usually require attention.

Think of gallstones as the starting point. Many other problems arise from their presence.

Biliary Colic – The First Clear Signal

For many patients, the first noticeable symptom is biliary colic.

This is the typical gallbladder attack:

Pain in the upper abdomen

Often after meals

Lasting from minutes to a few hours

At this stage:

The blockage is temporary

The stone moves

The pain settles

But this is usually the beginning, not the end.

Cholecystitis – When Inflammation Develops

If the blockage persists, the gallbladder becomes inflamed. This is called cholecystitis.

It may be:

Acute, sudden and more severe

Chronic, due to repeated irritation over time

Symptoms become more persistent, and medical treatment becomes more important.

Stones in the Bile Duct – A More Serious Situation

Sometimes stones move out of the gallbladder into the bile ducts.

This leads to:

Obstruction of bile flow

Jaundice

Abnormal blood tests

This condition affects the entire biliary system.

Infections and Complications

When bile flow is blocked, infection can develop.

Important complications include:

Cholangitis, infection of the bile ducts

Pancreatitis, inflammation of the pancreas

Guidance from the National Health Service emphasizes that these conditions require prompt treatment.

Diseases of the Gallbladder

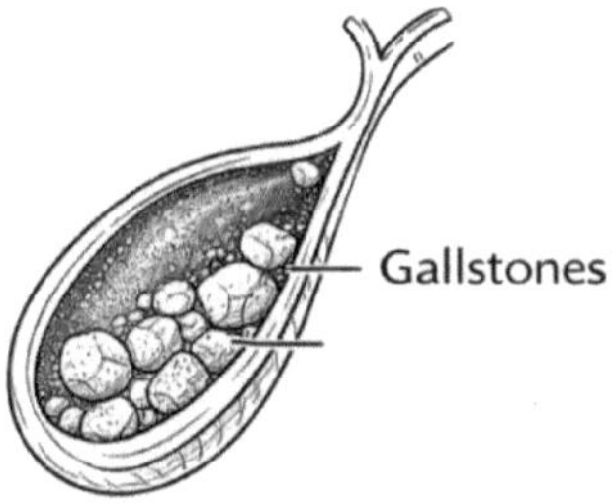

Gallstones
(Cholelithiasis)

Hardened deposits of cholesterol or bilirubin ↘ that form in the gallbladder.

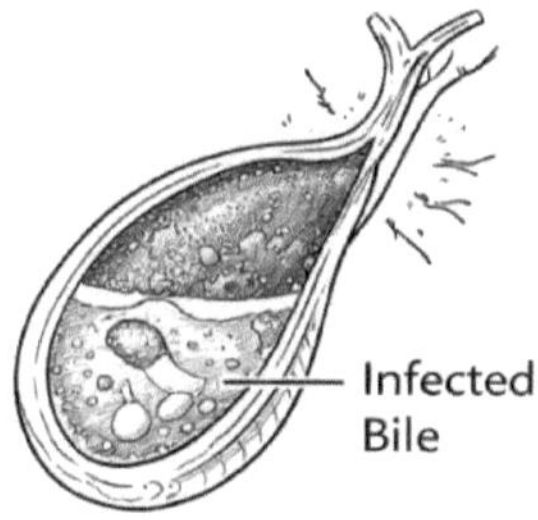

Gallbladder Infection
(Cholecystitis)

Inflammation of the gallbladder, often due to a blocked bile duct causing infection.

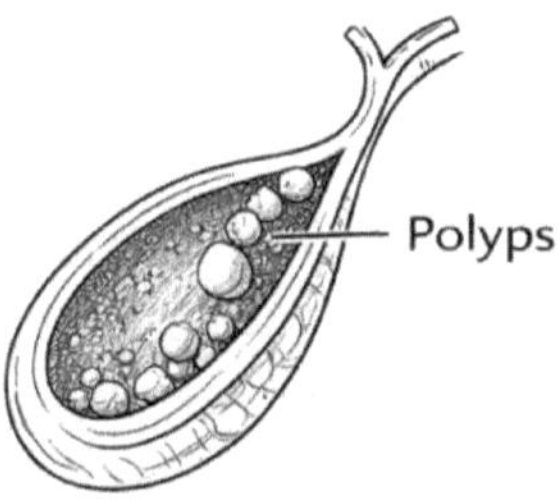

Gallbladder Polyps

Noncancerous growths that develop on the gallbladder wall

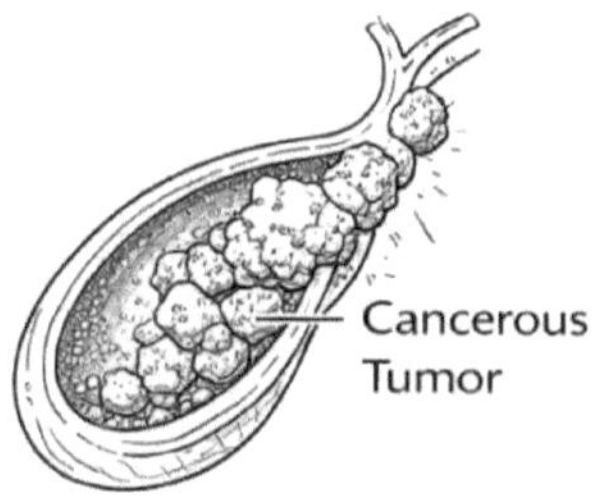

Gallbladder Cancer

A rare, but serious condition where malignant cells form in the gallbladder.

Gallstones can be made of hardened cholesterol, bilirubin, or a mix of both.

Functional Problems Without Stones

Not all gallbladder problems involve visible stones.

Some patients have:

Poor gallbladder emptying

Sludge or microscopic particles

Typical symptoms with normal imaging

These conditions can still cause real discomfort.

Polyps and Structural Changes

Imaging may sometimes show:

Polyps

Thickening of the gallbladder wall

Calcification

Most of these findings are harmless, but some require monitoring.

Rare but Important Conditions

Although uncommon, conditions such as gallbladder cancer are part of the overall picture.

It is important to be aware of them without becoming unnecessarily worried.

Why Symptoms Can Be Confusing

One challenge with gallbladder disease is that symptoms overlap with other conditions.

Pain in the upper abdomen may come from:

The stomach

The liver

The pancreas

Even the heart

This is why proper diagnosis is essential.

A Simple Way to Understand the Progression

In many patients, the sequence may look like this:

Stones form silently

Occasional pain begins

Pain becomes more frequent

Inflammation develops

Stones move into ducts

Complications may occur

Not everyone follows this exact path, but it is a helpful model.

Why This Chapter Matters

This chapter acts as a map.

When you understand the map:

Symptoms make more sense

Tests feel more logical

Treatment decisions become clearer

A Thought from My Practice

I often tell my patients that once they see the full picture, the condition feels less overwhelming and much more manageable.

Chapter Summary

Gallbladder disease includes a range of conditions, from silent gallstones to inflammation, bile duct obstruction, and complications such as infection and pancreatitis. Understanding this spectrum helps guide proper diagnosis and treatment.

Action Plan

If you have been diagnosed with gallstones, find out whether they are causing symptoms. Begin observing patterns carefully. Early understanding helps guide timely decisions.

Transition to Next Chapter

Now that you understand the full picture, we will focus on the most common issue in detail, gallstones, how they form, and why they behave differently in different people.

CHAPTER 4: Gallstones – What They Are and How They Form

Looking Closer at the Root of the Problem

Now that you understand the overall picture, it is time to focus on the most common cause of gallbladder disease, gallstones.

Many patients hear the term and imagine something large and fixed. In reality, gallstones vary widely. Some are tiny like grains of sand, while others can grow larger over time. Some remain silent for years, while others begin causing symptoms early.

Understanding what gallstones are and how they form makes everything else in this book easier to follow.

What Exactly Are Gallstones

Gallstones are solid particles that form from bile inside the gallbladder.

Bile is normally a liquid. But when its composition changes, certain substances come out of solution and form crystals. Over time, these crystals grow into stones.

A simple way to understand this is:

When too much of a substance is present, it begins to settle and form solid particles.

The Two Main Types of Gallstones

There are two main types.

Cholesterol stones: These are the most common, especially in the United States. They form when bile contains too much cholesterol and not enough substances to keep it dissolved.

Pigment stones: These are darker and form when there is excess bilirubin. They are more common in certain medical conditions.

According to the National Institute of Diabetes and Digestive and Kidney Diseases, cholesterol stones account for the majority of cases.

How Gallstones Form – Step by Step

Gallstones develop gradually over time.

The process can be understood in simple steps:

Imbalance in bile composition

Formation of small crystals

Growth and clustering of crystals

Poor emptying of the gallbladder

Development of larger stones

This slow progression explains why stones may exist long before symptoms begin.

Why Some Stones Cause Problems and Others Do Not

Many people have gallstones without symptoms.

Problems begin when:

Stones move

Stones block the outlet

Bile flow is interrupted

So the presence of stones alone is not the issue. Their behavior is what matters.

The Role of Gallbladder Function

The gallbladder actively contracts to release bile.

If it does not empty properly:

Bile becomes stagnant

Crystals have more time to form

Stones can grow

This is why reduced gallbladder activity increases risk.

Can Gallstones Disappear on Their Own

This is a common question.

In most cases, gallstones do not go away on their own.

Some medications may dissolve certain stones, but:

They work only in selected cases

They take a long time

Stones may return

For most patients, this is not a practical long-term solution.

What Happens If Gallstones Are Left Untreated

If stones are silent, they may never cause problems.

But once symptoms begin:

Episodes often recur

Pain may become more frequent

Risk of complications increases

This is why symptomatic gallstones require attention.

A Practical Way to Understand Gallstones

I often explain it simply:

Stones may remain quiet for years

When they begin to move, symptoms appear

Once symptoms start, they usually return

This pattern helps guide decisions.

Understanding Gallstones:
How Are They Formed?

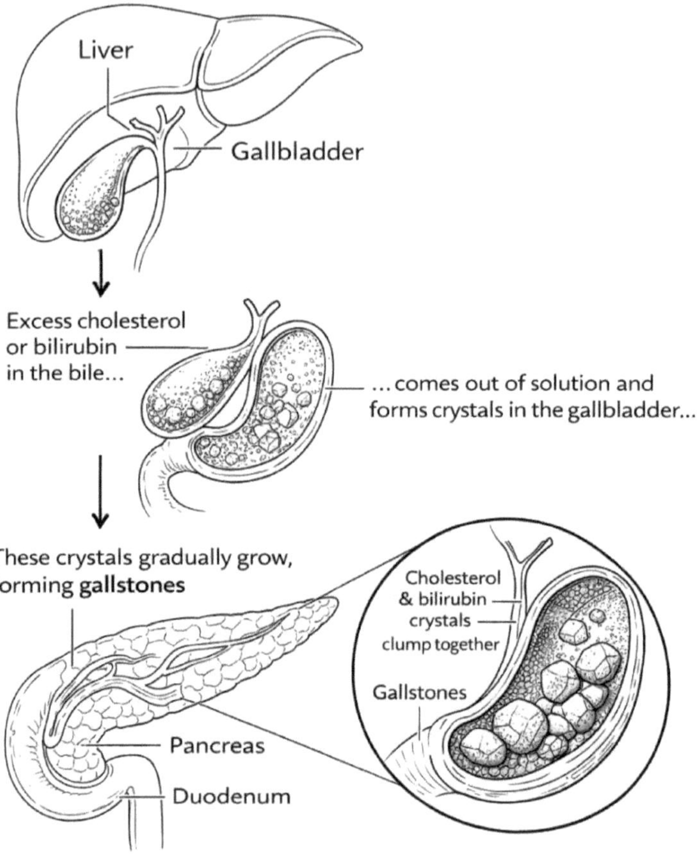

Gallstones can be made of hardened cholesterol, bilirubin, or a mix of both.

Why This Chapter Matters

Gallstones are the starting point for most gallbladder problems.

Understanding how they form and behave helps you:

Recognize symptoms

Understand diagnosis

Make informed treatment decisions

A Thought from My Practice

Patients often feel reassured when they understand that gallstones develop slowly and predictably. It makes the condition feel manageable rather than mysterious.

Chapter Summary

Gallstones form when bile becomes imbalanced and substances crystallize over time. Cholesterol stones are the most common. Many stones remain silent, but symptoms occur when they interfere with bile flow.

Action Plan

If you have gallstones, focus on whether they are causing symptoms. Observe patterns carefully. Do not assume they will disappear. Think in terms of long-term management.

Transition to Next Chapter

Now that you understand how gallstones form, the next step is to understand why they develop in some people and not in others.

CHAPTER 5: Why Gallstones Develop – Understanding Your Risk

A Question Almost Everyone Asks

Once gallstones are diagnosed, most patients ask:

"Why did this happen to me?"

It is a natural question. And the answer is important, not to assign blame, but to understand the condition and make better decisions going forward.

In most cases, there is no single cause. Gallstones develop over time due to a combination of factors. Some can be changed. Others cannot.

Understanding both gives you clarity and control.

The Most Important Risk Factor – Body Weight

Body weight plays a major role.

When body fat increases:

The liver produces more cholesterol

More cholesterol enters bile

The balance of bile is disturbed

This increases the chance of stone formation.

At the same time, an important point must be understood:

Rapid weight loss also increases risk.

During rapid weight loss:

The liver releases extra cholesterol

The gallbladder may not empty effectively

So both extremes, weight gain and rapid weight loss, can contribute.

Guidance from the National Institute of Diabetes and Digestive and Kidney Diseases highlights both as important risk factors.

Gender and Hormonal Influence

Gallstones are more common in women.

Hormones play a role:

Estrogen increases cholesterol in bile

It affects gallbladder movement

This is why gallstones are more often seen:

During pregnancy

With hormonal therapies

Age – Risk Increases Over Time

As age increases:

Bile composition changes

Gallbladder function may slow

This increases the likelihood of stone formation.

Many older adults have gallstones without symptoms.

Family History and Genetics

Some people have a natural tendency to develop gallstones.

If gallstones run in your family:

Your risk is higher

This does not guarantee that you will develop stones, but it is an important factor.

Diet – Important but Not the Only Factor

Diet plays a role, but it is often overemphasized.

Higher risk is associated with:

Diets rich in refined carbohydrates

Frequent intake of unhealthy fats

Lower risk is associated with:

Balanced meals

Adequate fiber intake

Diet is one factor among many.

Medical Conditions That Increase Risk

Certain conditions increase the likelihood of gallstones.

These include:

Diabetes

Liver disease

Conditions affecting red blood cells

These conditions influence bile composition and gallbladder function.

Medications and External Factors

Some medications can contribute to gallstone formation.

Examples include:

Hormonal medications

Certain cholesterol-related drugs

These effects are usually modest but worth noting.

The Combination Effect

One of the most important ideas is this:

Gallstones usually develop due to multiple factors acting together.

For example:

Genetic tendency

Weight changes

Hormonal influences

Eating patterns

This explains why different people have different risks.

What You Can Control

It is important to focus on what you can influence.

You can:

Maintain a healthy, stable weight

Avoid rapid weight loss

Follow a balanced diet

Stay physically active

Eat regular meals

These steps reduce risk and improve overall health.

What You Cannot Control

Some factors cannot be changed:

Age

Gender

Genetics

There is no benefit in worrying about these. Awareness is enough.

Why This Chapter Matters

Gallstones are not random.

They develop due to identifiable factors.

Understanding these factors helps you:

Reduce risk

Make better lifestyle choices

Feel more in control

A Thought from My Practice

I often tell my patients:

Do not focus on why this happened in the past. Focus on what you can improve from today.

Chapter Summary

Gallstones develop due to multiple factors including body weight, rapid weight loss, hormones, age, genetics, diet, and certain medical conditions. Some factors can be modified, while others cannot.

Action Plan

Review your own risk factors honestly. Aim for gradual and steady weight control. Avoid crash diets. Build simple, sustainable habits.

Transition to Next Chapter

Now that you understand why gallstones develop, the next step is to recognize how they present and how to identify early warning signs.

CHAPTER 6: Recognizing the Symptoms – When the Gallbladder Speaks

Why Early Signals Are Often Missed

One of the most common challenges in clinical practice is this:

The body gives signals, but they are often ignored in the beginning.

Gallbladder symptoms rarely start dramatically. They are usually subtle, easy to dismiss, and often mistaken for simple indigestion or gas.

A patient may say:
"I thought it was something I ate."
"I assumed it was acidity."

That is understandable. But when symptoms repeat in a pattern, they deserve attention.

The Most Common Symptom – Upper Abdominal Pain

The most important symptom of gallbladder disease is pain.

This pain is usually:

Felt in the upper right side of the abdomen

Sometimes in the middle upper abdomen

Deep, steady, and uncomfortable

It is not usually sharp or stabbing. Instead, it feels like a constant pressure or aching sensation.

Pain After Meals – A Key Clue

Timing is very important.

Gallbladder pain often:

Occurs after eating

Is more noticeable after fatty meals

Begins within minutes to a few hours

This happens because eating stimulates the gallbladder to contract. If a stone blocks the outlet, that contraction produces pain.

This pattern is one of the most helpful clues in diagnosis.

Pain That Spreads

Gallbladder pain does not always stay in one place.

It may spread to:

The right shoulder

The upper back

Between the shoulder blades

This can be confusing, and some patients initially think the pain is coming from their back.

Nausea and Digestive Discomfort

In addition to pain, many patients experience:

Nausea

Bloating

A feeling of fullness

These symptoms may occur with or without significant pain.

A Pattern of Episodes

In early stages, symptoms often follow a pattern:

Pain begins gradually

It builds in intensity

It lasts for a period

Then it settles

After the episode, the patient may feel completely normal.

This “come and go” pattern is typical.

When Symptoms Become More Serious

As the condition progresses, symptoms may change.

Warning signs include:

Pain lasting longer than usual

Increasing intensity

Fever

Persistent nausea or vomiting

General feeling of illness

These signs suggest inflammation or infection.

Jaundice – An Important Warning Sign

If a stone blocks the bile duct, bile cannot flow properly.

This may lead to:

Yellowing of the eyes and skin

Dark urine

Pale stools

This is called jaundice and requires prompt evaluation.

Guidance from the National Health Service emphasizes the importance of recognizing these symptoms early.

Symptoms That May Be Subtle

Not every patient presents with classic symptoms.

Some may have:

Mild discomfort

Occasional nausea

A general sense of digestive unease

These subtle symptoms still matter, especially if they repeat.

When It May Not Be the Gallbladder

Similar symptoms can arise from other conditions.

For example:

Acid reflux

Peptic ulcer disease

Pancreatic disorders

This is why proper evaluation is important.

Listening to Patterns

One of the most useful steps you can take is observing patterns.

Ask yourself:

When does the pain occur

What triggers it

How long it lasts

Whether it repeats

These observations help guide diagnosis.

Symptoms of Gallbladder Disease

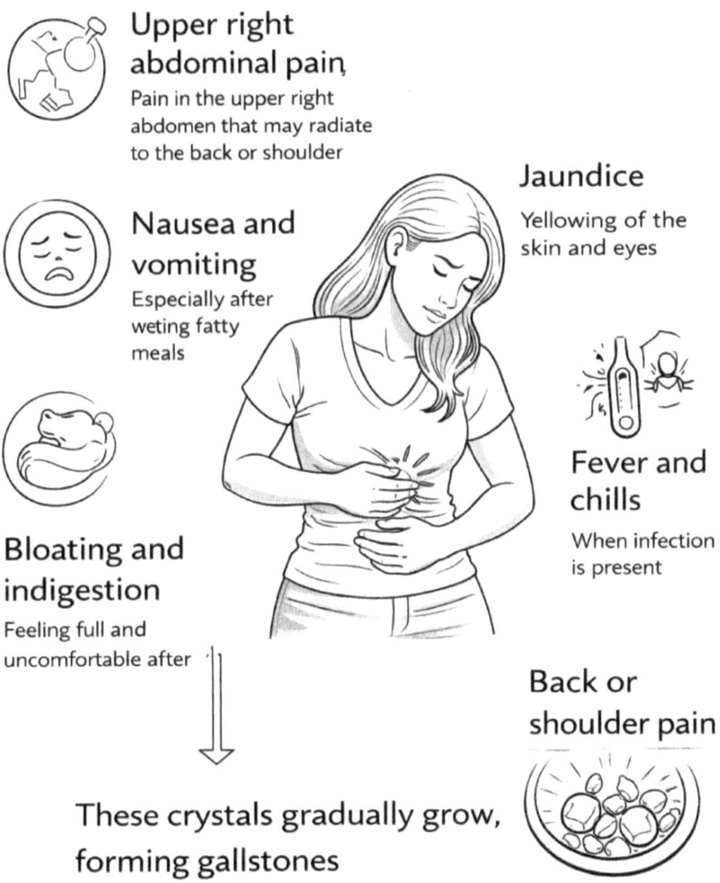

A Thought from My Practice

I often tell my patients:

A single episode may not mean much. But repeated patterns usually mean something.

Chapter Summary

Gallbladder disease commonly presents with upper abdominal pain, especially after meals. Pain may spread to the back or shoulder and may be associated with nausea and bloating. Early symptoms are often intermittent but should not be ignored.

Action Plan

Pay attention to recurring symptoms, especially after meals. Note patterns carefully. Seek medical advice if symptoms persist or worsen.

Transition to Next Chapter

Now that you understand the symptoms, the next step is to recognize the most typical presentation in detail, the classic gallbladder attack.

CHAPTER 7: Biliary Colic – The Classic Gallbladder Attack

When the Gallbladder Finally Gets Your Attention

Up to this point, symptoms may have been mild or uncertain.

Then comes an episode that feels different.

Many patients describe it as the moment they realize something is not quite right. The discomfort is stronger, more focused, and harder to ignore.

This is what we call **biliary colic**, the typical gallbladder attack.

Understanding What Is Happening Inside

After you eat, especially a fatty meal, the gallbladder contracts to release bile.

If a stone is present near the outlet:

It may temporarily block the flow

The gallbladder continues to contract

Pressure builds up

Pain begins and gradually increases

After some time:

The stone may shift

The blockage clears

Pressure reduces

Pain settles

This explains why the attack eventually passes.

How the Pain Feels

Patients describe this pain in consistent ways.

The pain is usually:

Located in the upper right or middle upper abdomen

Deep, steady, and often intense

Not relieved by changing position

Lasting from about 30 minutes to a few hours

It typically builds up, reaches a steady level, and then gradually fades.

According to the National Institute of Diabetes and Digestive and Kidney Diseases, this is the classic pattern.

Pain That Travels

One important feature is that the pain may spread.

It can radiate to:

The right shoulder

The upper back

Between the shoulder blades

This often confuses patients.

Common Triggers

There is often a relationship with food.

Common triggers include:

Fried or greasy meals

Heavy meals after a long gap

Rich, high-fat foods

However, not every episode follows a heavy meal.

How Long Does an Attack Last

A typical episode:

Begins gradually

Builds in intensity

Lasts for a few hours

Then settles

If pain lasts much longer or continues to worsen, it may not be simple biliary colic.

What Happens Between Attacks

Between episodes, most patients feel completely normal.

This can be misleading.

A person may think the problem has gone away. But the underlying issue remains.

Over time:

Episodes may become stronger

Attacks may occur more frequently

How It Differs from Acidity or Gas

Biliary colic is often mistaken for acidity.

Key differences include:

Pain is steady, not burning

It does not improve with antacids

It is often related to meals

It may spread to the back or shoulder

When It Is No Longer Just an Attack

Be alert to changes in the pattern.

Seek medical attention if you notice:

Pain lasting longer than usual

Increasing severity

Fever

Persistent vomiting

A general feeling of illness

These suggest progression.

Why Repeated Attacks Matter

Each episode is a signal.

Repeated attacks indicate:

Stones are active

The gallbladder is under stress

Risk of complications is increasing

Ignoring repeated episodes may lead to more serious problems.

What You Should Do During an Episode

During an attack:

Rest

Avoid further food intake

Observe duration and intensity

Seek medical advice if:

It is your first episode

Pain is severe, or attacks are recurring

A Thought from My Practice

I often tell my patients:

The first attack is a warning. Repeated attacks are a pattern. Patterns should not be ignored.

Chapter Summary

Biliary colic is the typical gallbladder attack caused by temporary blockage of bile flow. It presents as steady upper abdominal pain, often after meals, lasting for a few hours and then resolving.

Action Plan

If you experience this pattern, track episodes carefully. Note timing, triggers, and duration. Seek medical evaluation early.

Transition to Next Chapter

Now that you understand the typical gallbladder attack, the next step is to recognize when the condition progresses to inflammation.

CHAPTER 8: Cholecystitis – When Inflammation Changes the Situation

When the Pattern Shifts

Until now, we have been discussing pain that comes and goes.

Cholecystitis is different.

This is the point where the pattern changes. The pain no longer settles quickly. The body begins to react more strongly. What started as a temporary blockage becomes a sustained problem.

In simple terms:

Biliary colic is a warning

Cholecystitis is progression

Recognizing this shift is very important.

What Exactly Is Cholecystitis

Cholecystitis means inflammation of the gallbladder.

It usually occurs when:

A gallstone blocks the cystic duct

Bile cannot leave the gallbladder

Pressure builds up

The gallbladder wall becomes inflamed

In some cases, bacteria grow in the trapped bile, leading to infection.

According to the National Institute of Diabetes and Digestive and Kidney Diseases, this is the most common cause.

Acute Cholecystitis – Sudden and More Severe

Acute cholecystitis develops quickly.

Common features include:

Persistent upper right abdominal pain

Pain lasting longer than a few hours

Fever

Nausea and vomiting

Tenderness on examination

Patients often say:
"This feels different from my earlier attacks."

That difference is important.

Chronic Cholecystitis – A Slower Process

Chronic cholecystitis develops over time due to repeated irritation.

It may present with:

Recurrent discomfort after meals

Less intense but frequent pain

Ongoing digestive symptoms

The gallbladder gradually becomes less effective.

How It Differs from Biliary Colic

It helps to see the difference clearly.

Biliary colic:

Pain comes and goes

No fever

Normal feeling between episodes

Cholecystitis:

Pain persists

Fever may be present

General feeling of illness

How Doctors Make the Diagnosis

Diagnosis is based on a combination of findings.

Doctors look for:

Persistent symptoms

Tenderness on examination

Signs of inflammation in blood tests

Changes on ultrasound

Why Early Treatment Matters

If untreated, complications can develop.

These may include:

Severe infection

Pus formation

Rupture of the gallbladder

Spread of infection

Early treatment helps prevent these outcomes.

How It Is Treated

Treatment usually begins in the hospital.

It may include:

Intravenous fluids

Pain control

Antibiotics if infection is present

In many cases, surgery is recommended during the same admission or soon after recovery.

A Simple Way to Understand It

I often explain it simply:

If the stone moves, you get pain.
If the stone stays, you get inflammation.

When You Should Be Concerned

Take symptoms seriously if you notice:

Pain lasting longer than usual

Fever

Persistent nausea or vomiting

Feeling unwell

These suggest progression.

A Thought from My Practice

Many patients sense that something is different but delay seeking care. Acting early often makes a significant difference.

Chapter Summary

Cholecystitis is inflammation of the gallbladder caused by persistent blockage, usually from a gallstone. It presents with continuous pain, fever, and signs of illness. Early treatment is important.

Action Plan

If you experience persistent pain, especially with fever or nausea, seek medical care promptly. Do not assume it will settle on its own.

Transition to Next Chapter

Now that you understand gallbladder inflammation, the next step is to see what happens when stones move beyond the gallbladder into the bile ducts.

CHAPTER 9: When Stones Move – Stones in the Bile Duct (Choledocholithiasis)

When the Problem Extends Beyond the Gallbladder

So far, we have focused on what happens inside the gallbladder.

But sometimes, the situation does not stay confined there.

A stone can move out of the gallbladder and enter the bile duct. When this happens, the problem becomes more serious because the bile duct is the main pathway through which bile flows from the liver into the intestine.

This condition is called choledocholithiasis, or stones in the bile duct.

Why This Is More Serious

The gallbladder stores bile, but the bile duct carries it.

When a stone blocks the gallbladder:

You feel pain

When a stone blocks the bile duct:

The entire system is affected

This leads to:

Blocked bile flow

Pressure buildup in the liver

Accumulation of waste products in the blood

That is why bile duct stones require more urgent attention.

How Stones Reach the Bile Duct

Most bile duct stones begin in the gallbladder.

They:

Form in the gallbladder

Travel through the cystic duct

Enter the common bile duct

Less commonly, stones can form directly in the bile duct.

Recognizing the Symptoms

Symptoms often differ from simple gallbladder pain.

Common features include:

Upper abdominal pain

Jaundice, yellowing of the eyes and skin

Dark urine

Pale stools

Itching

According to the National Health Service, these are key signs of bile duct obstruction.

Understanding Jaundice Clearly

Jaundice is an important sign.

When bile flow is blocked:

Bilirubin builds up in the blood

Skin and eyes turn yellow

Urine becomes dark

Stools become pale

This always requires medical attention.

What Blood Tests Show

Blood tests provide important clues.

Doctors may find:

Elevated bilirubin

Increased liver enzymes

Signs of bile duct obstruction

These results indicate the problem is beyond the gallbladder.

How the Diagnosis Is Confirmed

Imaging is essential.

Tests may include:

Ultrasound

MRCP

Endoscopic ultrasound

These help locate the stone and assess the blockage.

ERCP – A Key Treatment Tool

One of the most important procedures is ERCP.

It allows doctors to:

Locate the stone

Remove it

Relieve the blockage

This procedure both diagnoses and treats the condition.

Why Timely Treatment Matters

Delaying treatment can lead to complications such as:

Infection of the bile ducts

Pancreatitis

Liver-related problems

Early treatment prevents these outcomes.

What Happens After Treatment

After removing the bile duct stone:

The gallbladder is usually treated as well

If gallstones remain:

Surgery is often recommended

This prevents recurrence.

A Simple Way to Understand It

I often explain it like this:

Gallbladder stones cause pain.
Bile duct stones affect the whole system.

When to Seek Immediate Care

Seek urgent care if you notice:

Yellowing of the eyes or skin

Dark urine or pale stools

Persistent abdominal pain

These are important warning signs.

A Thought from My Practice

Patients who recognize jaundice early and seek care promptly usually recover more smoothly.

Chapter Summary

Bile duct stones occur when gallstones move into the common bile duct and block bile flow. This leads to jaundice, abnormal blood tests, and risk of complications. Treatment often involves ERCP.

Action Plan

If you notice jaundice or related symptoms, seek medical care immediately. Follow recommended tests and treatment plans carefully.

Transition to Next Chapter

Now that you understand bile duct stones, the next step is to recognize serious complications that can arise from them.

CHAPTER 10: When Things Turn Serious – Cholangitis and Gallstone Pancreatitis

A Turning Point You Should Recognize

Up to now, we have discussed pain, inflammation, and blockage. Most of these situations, though uncomfortable, are manageable.

But there is a point where the condition can become urgent.

In real-life practice, the difference is often how quickly things change. What was once a recurring problem suddenly becomes more intense, more persistent, and is accompanied by new symptoms.

Two conditions deserve special attention:

Cholangitis, an infection of the bile ducts

Gallstone pancreatitis, inflammation of the pancreas

Recognizing these early can make a critical difference.

Cholangitis – Infection Behind a Blockage

Cholangitis occurs when a bile duct is blocked and bacteria grow in stagnant bile.

The sequence is simple:

A stone blocks the bile duct

Bile cannot flow

Bacteria multiply

Infection develops

Because the bile ducts connect to the bloodstream, infection can spread quickly.

This makes cholangitis a medical emergency.

The Typical Symptoms of Cholangitis

There is a well-known combination of symptoms:

Fever with chills

Abdominal pain

Jaundice

Not every patient has all three, but when they occur together, they strongly suggest cholangitis.

Other symptoms may include:

Weakness

Nausea and vomiting

Confusion, especially in older adults

Guidance from the National Health Service emphasizes the need for urgent evaluation.

Why Cholangitis Is Dangerous

The danger lies in the spread of infection.

If not treated promptly:

Bacteria can enter the bloodstream

Sepsis can develop

Blood pressure may fall

Multiple organs may be affected

Immediate treatment is essential.

How Cholangitis Is Treated

Treatment has two key parts:

First, control the infection:

Hospital admission

Intravenous antibiotics

Supportive care

Second, relieve the blockage:

Usually with ERCP

Drainage of bile

Removal of the stone

Both steps are necessary.

Gallstone Pancreatitis – When the Pancreas Is Involved

The bile duct and pancreatic duct meet before entering the intestine.

If a stone gets stuck at this junction:

It can block both ducts

This can trigger pancreatitis

This condition is called gallstone pancreatitis.

Symptoms of Gallstone Pancreatitis

This condition often presents with:

Severe upper abdominal pain

Pain radiating to the back

Persistent nausea and vomiting

Inability to tolerate food

The pain is usually continuous and more intense than biliary colic.

How Serious Is Pancreatitis

Pancreatitis can vary in severity.

In mild cases:

Recovery occurs with supportive care

In more severe cases:

Complications may develop

Intensive care may be required

Recovery may take longer

Information from the National Institute of Diabetes and Digestive and Kidney Diseases highlights the need for careful monitoring.

How It Is Treated

Treatment usually includes:

Hospital care

Intravenous fluids

Pain control

Temporary rest for digestion

If a bile duct stone is present:

It may need to be removed

After recovery:

Gallbladder removal is often recommended

Cholangitis and Pancreatitis

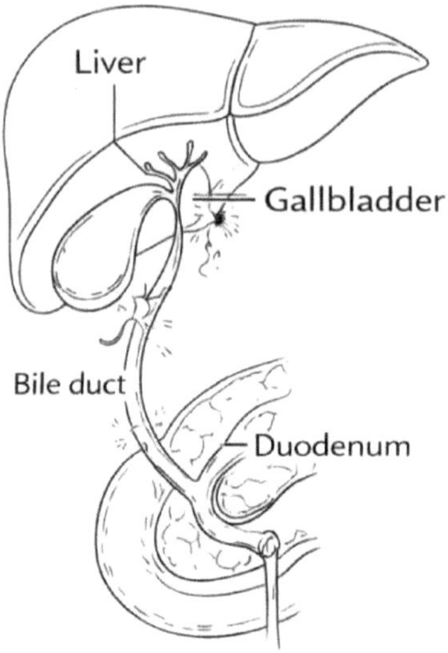

Cholangitis

Infection and inflammation of the bile ducts, often due to a gallstone blocking the duct, leading to pus buildup.

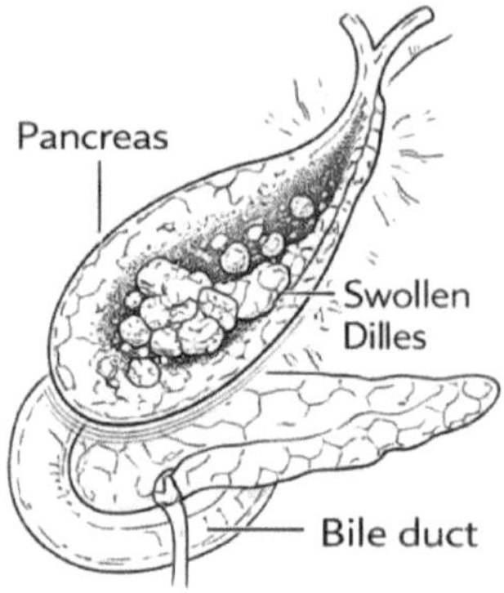

Pancreatitis

Inflammation of the pancreas, often due to gallstones blocking the panceratic duct or issues with digestion of digestive enzymes.

How These Conditions Are Connected

It helps to see the sequence clearly:

Gallstones form in the gallbladder

A stone moves into the bile duct

The duct becomes blocked

From here:

Infection develops → cholangitis

Or pancreatic inflammation occurs → pancreatitis

Warning Signs You Should Never Ignore

Seek immediate medical care if you have:

Fever with abdominal pain

Yellowing of the eyes or skin

Severe, persistent abdominal pain

Repeated vomiting

Weakness or confusion

These require urgent attention.

A Thought from My Practice

In many cases, the difference between a smooth recovery and a complicated one is how early care is sought.

Chapter Summary

Cholangitis is a serious infection of the bile ducts, and gallstone pancreatitis is inflammation of the pancreas caused by stones. Both arise from bile duct blockage and require urgent medical treatment.

Action Plan

If you develop fever, jaundice, or severe persistent pain, seek emergency care immediately. Do not delay.

Transition to Next Chapter

Now that you understand serious complications, the next step is to explore conditions where symptoms occur even without visible stones.

CHAPTER 11: When Tests Are Normal but Symptoms Persist – Functional Gallbladder Disorders

A Situation That Can Be Frustrating

By this point, you may expect that every gallbladder problem shows up clearly on a scan.

In real life, that is not always the case.

I have seen many patients with typical symptoms, pain after meals, upper abdominal discomfort, nausea, yet their ultrasound report looks normal. No stones.

Naturally, this creates confusion.

"If everything is normal, why do I still feel this way?"

This is where we need to look beyond what is visible.

The Idea of Function, Not Just Structure

Most people think of disease as something structural, something that can be seen.

But some problems are functional.

This means:

The gallbladder is present

There are no visible stones

But it does not function properly

In these cases, the issue is not structure. It is function.

Biliary Dyskinesia – Poor Gallbladder Emptying

One of the key conditions in this group is biliary dyskinesia.

In simple terms:

The gallbladder does not contract effectively

Bile is not released properly

Pressure builds up and causes symptoms

Symptoms often resemble gallstone disease:

Pain after meals

Upper abdominal discomfort

Nausea

Feeling of fullness

How This Condition Is Evaluated

When ultrasound is normal but symptoms suggest gallbladder disease, a HIDA scan may be recommended.

This test evaluates:

Entry of bile into the gallbladder

How well the gallbladder empties

A low ejection fraction suggests poor gallbladder function.

Sludge and Microscopic Stones

Sometimes the issue is not absence of stones, but stones too small to be clearly seen.

These include:

Sludge

Microscopic stones

They can still:

Interfere with bile flow

Cause symptoms

Lead to inflammation

In some cases, sludge resolves. In others, it progresses to stones.

Acalculous Cholecystitis

Another condition is inflammation without stones.

This is called acalculous cholecystitis.

It is more common in:

Critically ill patients

Hospitalized individuals

But milder forms can occur.

Why Diagnosis Can Be Challenging

These conditions are more difficult to diagnose because:

Imaging may appear normal

Symptoms overlap with other conditions

There is no single definitive test

Clinical judgment becomes very important.

How Doctors Approach These Cases

A thoughtful approach includes:

Careful review of symptoms

Attention to meal-related patterns

Additional testing when needed

Excluding other causes

The goal is accuracy, not speed.

When Treatment May Still Be Needed

Even without visible stones, treatment may be considered if:

Symptoms are persistent

Daily life is affected

Functional tests show abnormality

In selected cases, surgery may provide relief.

Avoiding Common Mistakes

Two common mistakes are:

Ignoring symptoms because tests are normal

Proceeding to surgery without proper evaluation

A balanced approach is essential.

The Importance of Patterns

Patterns are especially important here.

If you notice:

Repeated symptoms

Clear relation to meals

Similar episodes over time

then further evaluation is justified.

A Thought from My Practice

I often tell my patients:

Normal tests do not always mean nothing is wrong. Sometimes we need to look deeper.

Chapter Summary

Some gallbladder problems occur without visible stones. Conditions such as biliary dyskinesia, sludge, and acalculous cholecystitis can cause symptoms despite normal imaging.

Action Plan

If symptoms persist despite normal tests, do not ignore them. Track patterns and discuss further evaluation with your doctor.

Transition to Next Chapter

Now that we have explored functional disorders, the next step is to understand findings that appear on imaging and what they really mean.

CHAPTER 12: Gallbladder Polyps and Incidental Findings- What They Mean & When to Act

When a Report Creates More Questions Than Answers

This is a situation I see very often.

A patient undergoes an ultrasound, sometimes for routine reasons, and the report mentions something unexpected. Words like "polyp," "wall thickening," or "sludge" appear.

The immediate reaction is understandable:
"Is this serious?"
"Do I need surgery?"

In many cases, the answer is reassuring. But not always. The key is to understand what these findings actually mean.

Gallbladder Polyps – Usually Harmless

Gallbladder polyps are small growths from the inner lining of the gallbladder.

Most polyps are:

Small

Benign

Discovered incidentally

They usually do not cause symptoms and are often unrelated to the pain a patient may be experiencing.

Guidance from the National Health Service indicates that most gallbladder polyps are not dangerous.

Size Matters – A Practical Way to Think About It

When it comes to polyps, size is important.

In general:

Very small polyps are usually harmless

Larger polyps need closer observation

Growth over time is significant

Doctors often recommend monitoring rather than immediate surgery for small, stable polyps.

When Polyps Need Closer Attention

Further evaluation may be needed if:

The polyp is larger than expected

It increases in size

There are additional risk factors

Symptoms are present

In such situations, surgical consultation may be advised.

Gallbladder Wall Thickening

Another common finding is thickening of the gallbladder wall.

This can occur due to:

Acute inflammation

Chronic irritation

Temporary conditions such as infection or fluid changes

It does not always indicate a serious problem. Context matters.

Gallbladder Sludge – An Early Stage

Sometimes the report mentions sludge.

This refers to thickened bile containing tiny particles.

Sludge can:

Resolve on its own

Cause symptoms similar to stones

Progress to gallstones

Management depends on symptoms and follow-up.

Porcelain Gallbladder – A Rare but Important Finding

Porcelain gallbladder refers to calcification of the gallbladder wall.

It is uncommon but important.

It is usually associated with:

Long-standing inflammation

Chronic gallbladder disease

It may require closer evaluation and sometimes surgery.

When Findings Do Not Match Symptoms

Sometimes:

The report shows findings, but you have no symptoms

Or you have symptoms, but the report is minimal

This can be confusing.

Treatment decisions depend on:

Symptoms

Risk factors

Overall clinical picture

Avoiding Unnecessary Fear

Not every abnormal finding is serious.

Many findings are:

Incidental

Stable

Not harmful

At the same time, some require attention. Balance is important.

How Doctors Decide What to Do

Doctors consider:

Size and appearance

Presence of symptoms

Changes over time

Overall health

Based on this, they may recommend:

Observation

Repeat imaging

Further testing

Surgery

A Practical Way to Approach Your Report

When you receive a report:

Do not panic

Focus on the summary

Avoid over-interpreting details

Discuss it with your doctor

A Thought from My Practice

Many patients feel anxious reading reports alone. A simple discussion often brings clarity and relief.

Chapter Summary

Gallbladder imaging may reveal polyps, sludge, or wall thickening. Most findings are benign and require monitoring rather than immediate treatment.

Action Plan

If your report shows any finding, discuss it calmly with your doctor. Follow recommended follow-up. Avoid unnecessary anxiety.

Transition to Next Chapter

Now that we have discussed incidental findings, the next step is to understand a rare but important condition, gallbladder cancer.

CHAPTER 13: Gallbladder Cancer – Awareness Without Unnecessary Fear

A Topic That Needs Clarity, Not Anxiety

At some point, almost every patient with gallbladder disease asks:

"Could this be cancer?"

It is a natural concern. The word itself can create fear even when the actual risk is low.

Let me reassure you clearly:

Gallbladder cancer is rare.

Most people with gallstones or gallbladder symptoms will never develop cancer. Still, it is important to understand this condition calmly and realistically.

How Common Is It

Compared to other digestive cancers, gallbladder cancer is uncommon.

However, it is important because:

It is often detected late

Early symptoms are not very specific

Early detection improves outcomes

Information from the National Cancer Institute confirms that while the disease is rare, awareness is important.

Who Is at Higher Risk

Most people are at low risk, but certain factors increase the likelihood.

These include:

Long-standing gallstones

Chronic inflammation

Porcelain gallbladder

Larger gallbladder polyps

Increasing age

Certain genetic and geographic factors

Having gallstones does not mean you will develop cancer.

The Role of Long-Term Inflammation

One of the key links is chronic irritation.

Over time:

Repeated inflammation can damage the lining

Cells may undergo gradual changes

This may increase the risk of abnormal growth

This is why long-standing disease is monitored more carefully.

Early Symptoms – Often Vague

Early symptoms are not specific.

They may include:

Mild upper abdominal discomfort

Indigestion-like symptoms

Occasional nausea

These overlap with common digestive problems.

Symptoms in More Advanced Stages

As the condition progresses, symptoms may become more noticeable:

Persistent abdominal pain

Unexplained weight loss

Jaundice

Loss of appetite

General weakness

These often appear later in the disease.

How It Is Detected

Gallbladder cancer is often found:

Incidentally on imaging

During surgery for gallstones

During evaluation of persistent symptoms

Ultrasound, CT scan, or MRI may raise suspicion.

Diagnosis and Evaluation

If cancer is suspected, doctors may recommend:

Detailed imaging

Blood tests

Biopsy in selected cases

The stage of the disease is then determined.

Treatment Options

Treatment depends on stage.

In early stages:

Surgery may be curative

In advanced stages:

Additional surgery

Chemotherapy or other treatments

Each case is individualized.

Why Routine Screening Is Not Common

Routine screening is not widely done because:

The disease is rare

There is no simple screening test

Focus is placed on high-risk individuals.

A Reassuring Perspective

In practice, gallbladder cancer is uncommon.

For most patients:

The risk is low

Proper management reduces risk

Awareness is sufficient

There is no need for constant worry.

When You Should Be More Alert

Seek evaluation if:

You have long-standing disease

You have been told about large polyps

You develop unexplained weight loss, or symptoms become persistent

---

A Thought from My Practice

I often tell my patients:

Know about it, but do not fear it. Awareness helps you act wisely if needed.

Chapter Summary

Gallbladder cancer is rare but important. It is associated with long-standing disease and chronic inflammation. Early symptoms are subtle, and awareness is key.

Action Plan

Do not assume gallstones mean cancer. Follow up on significant findings. Seek advice for persistent symptoms. Stay informed without anxiety.

Transition to Next Chapter

Now that we have covered gallbladder-specific conditions, the next step is to understand other conditions that can mimic similar symptoms.

CHAPTER 14: When It Is Not the Gallbladder – Conditions That Mimic Gallbladder Disease

Why Getting the Diagnosis Right Matters

By now, you understand how gallbladder disease presents.

But in real clinical practice, not every upper abdominal pain comes from the gallbladder.

I have seen patients convinced they have gallbladder disease when the cause was something else. I have also seen the opposite, patients treating what they thought was simple acidity when the gallbladder was the real issue.

This overlap makes accurate diagnosis essential.

Why So Many Conditions Feel Similar

The upper abdomen is a complex area.

Several important organs are located close together:

Stomach

Liver

Gallbladder

Pancreas

Intestine

Because of this:

Pain from different organs can feel similar

Symptoms can overlap

Location alone is not enough for diagnosis

Doctors rely on patterns rather than a single symptom.

Acid Reflux and Peptic Ulcer Disease

One of the most common mimics is acid-related disease.

This includes:

Acid reflux

Peptic ulcers

Symptoms may include:

Burning discomfort

Pain related to meals

Relief with antacids

Key differences:

Pain is often burning

It may improve with medication

It is less specifically related to fatty meals

Information from the National Institute of Diabetes and Digestive and Kidney Diseases supports these patterns.

Liver Conditions

The liver lies close to the gallbladder.

Conditions such as:

Hepatitis

Fatty liver disease

may cause:

Dull right-sided discomfort

Fatigue

Abnormal blood tests

This discomfort is usually less intense and not episodic.

Pancreatic Disorders

The pancreas is closely connected to the bile system.

Conditions like pancreatitis may present with:

Severe upper abdominal pain

Pain radiating to the back

Persistent symptoms

Pain is usually continuous and more severe.

Irritable Bowel Syndrome and Functional Disorders

Functional disorders may also overlap.

Symptoms include:

Bloating

Abdominal discomfort

Changes in bowel habits

The presence of bowel changes helps distinguish these from gallbladder disease.

Kidney Stones

Kidney stones can sometimes mimic gallbladder pain.

Typical features include:

Pain starting in the back or flank

Pain that moves forward

Severe, wave-like discomfort

Urinary symptoms may also be present.

Heart-Related Conditions

This is an important point.

In some patients, especially older adults, heart conditions may present with upper abdominal discomfort.

Symptoms may include:

Pressure in the chest or upper abdomen

Shortness of breath

Pain radiating to the arm

This is why doctors sometimes evaluate the heart.

Musculoskeletal Pain

Pain from muscles or the chest wall may also mimic internal problems.

This type of pain:

Is localized

Worsens with movement or touch

Is not related to meals

How Doctors Tell the Difference

Doctors consider:

Pattern of pain

Timing with meals

Associated symptoms

Blood tests and imaging

These together help identify the cause.

Your Role in the Process

You can help by:

Describing symptoms clearly

Noting patterns

Reporting associated symptoms

Clear communication improves accuracy.

A Thought from My Practice

I often tell my patients not to rely on a single symptom. The pattern over time tells the real story.

Chapter Summary

Many conditions can mimic gallbladder disease, including acid reflux, liver disease, pancreatic disorders, IBS, kidney stones, and heart conditions. Accurate diagnosis depends on recognizing patterns.

Action Plan

Avoid self-diagnosis. Track your symptoms and triggers. Seek medical evaluation when symptoms are persistent or unclear.

Transition to Next Chapter

Now that you understand symptom overlap, the next step is to see how doctors arrive at the correct diagnosis using tests and imaging.

CHAPTER 15: How Doctors Make the Diagnosis – A Clear, Step-by-Step Approach

Diagnosis Is Built, Not Found in One Test

Many patients expect one test to give a clear answer.

In reality, diagnosis is a step-by-step process. It is built using different pieces of information that come together to form a complete picture.

These include:

Your symptoms

Physical examination

Blood tests

Imaging

When interpreted together, they provide clarity.

Step 1: Listening to Your Story

The most important step often begins with a careful discussion.

Doctors ask:

Where is the pain

When does it occur

Is it related to meals

How long does it last

What makes it better or worse

These details are extremely valuable.

Pain after fatty meals, for example, strongly suggests gallbladder involvement.

Step 2: Physical Examination

Next comes examination.

Doctors look for:

Tenderness in the upper right abdomen

Pain on pressure

Signs of inflammation

Sometimes pressing under the right rib during deep breathing causes discomfort. This can be an important clue.

Step 3: Blood Tests – What They Show

Blood tests do not show gallstones directly, but they provide important information.

They help detect:

Infection or inflammation

Liver involvement

Bile duct obstruction

Pancreatic involvement

Common findings include:

Elevated white blood cell count

Increased bilirubin

Elevated liver enzymes

Raised pancreatic enzymes

Step 4: Ultrasound – The First and Most Important Test

Ultrasound is usually the first imaging test.

It is:

Safe

Non-invasive

Widely available

It can detect:

Gallstones

Gallbladder wall thickening

Signs of inflammation

Dilated bile ducts

According to the National Institute of Diabetes and Digestive and Kidney Diseases, ultrasound is the preferred initial test.

Step 5: HIDA Scan – Checking Function

If symptoms are typical but ultrasound is normal, a HIDA scan may be recommended.

It evaluates:

Entry of bile into the gallbladder

How well the gallbladder empties

A low ejection fraction suggests poor function.

Step 6: CT Scan and MRI – A Broader View

When more detail is needed, additional imaging is used.

CT scan helps:

Evaluate complications

Assess surrounding organs

MRI helps:

Visualize bile ducts

Detect obstruction

Step 7: MRCP – A Focused Look at the Bile Ducts

MRCP is a specialized MRI technique.

It allows doctors to:

See bile ducts clearly

Identify stones or blockages

Plan treatment

It is non-invasive and highly informative.

Step 8: Endoscopic Ultrasound

In selected cases, endoscopic ultrasound is used.

It combines:

Endoscopy

Ultrasound

It provides detailed imaging, especially for small stones.

Step 9: ERCP – Diagnosis and Treatment Together

ERCP is used when intervention is required.

It allows doctors to:

Identify stones in the bile duct

Remove them.

Relieve obstruction

It is usually performed when treatment is needed.

Putting It All Together

Diagnosis is not based on one test.

Doctors combine:

Symptoms

Examination findings

Blood tests

Imaging

Each part contributes to the final diagnosis.

When the Diagnosis Is Not Immediately Clear

Sometimes:

Symptoms are present

Tests are inconclusive

In such cases:

Doctors may monitor

Repeat tests

Consider other causes

Patience is important.

Diagnosing Gallbladder Disease

How Diagnosis Is Made

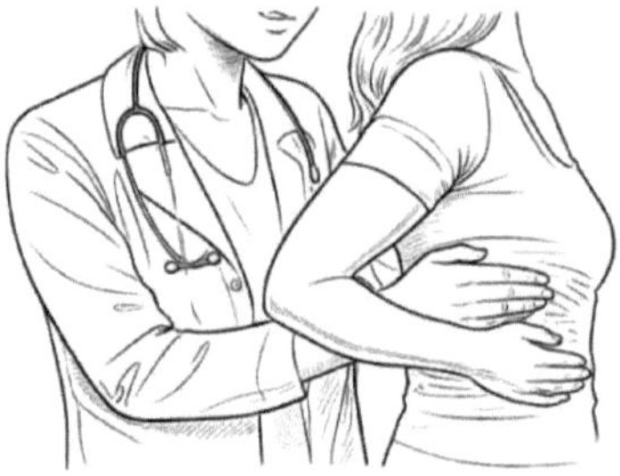

Physical Examination

Doctor checks for tenderness in the upper right abdomen and notes symptoms.

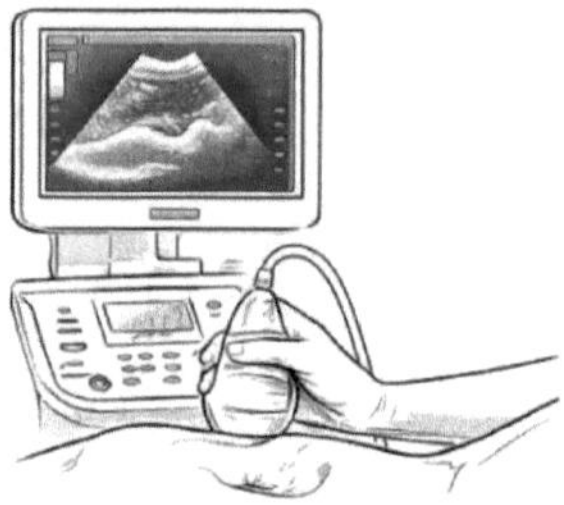

Ultrasound (Sonogram)

Uses sound waves to create images of the gallbladder and bile ducts

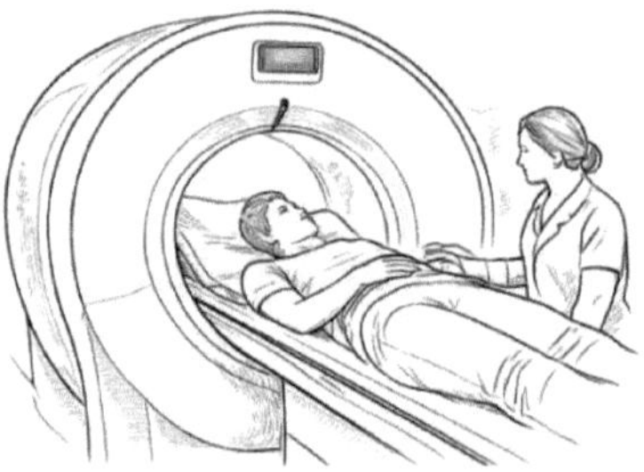

MRI / CT Scan

Produces detailed cross-sectional images of the gallbladder and surrounding organs

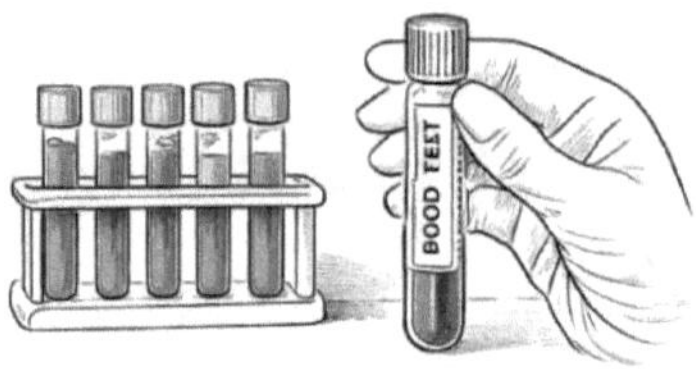

Blood Tests

Check liver function, signs of infection, or inflammation

Your Role in the Process

You play a key role.

You can help by:

Describing symptoms clearly

Keeping track of patterns

Following through with tests

A Thought from My Practice

I often tell my patients:

Do not look for one test to give all the answers. Look at the complete picture.

Chapter Summary

Diagnosis of gallbladder disease involves a structured approach using history, examination, blood tests, and imaging. Ultrasound is the first test, followed by other investigations when needed.

Action Plan

Be prepared to describe your symptoms clearly. Follow your doctor's advice regarding tests. Stay patient as the diagnosis becomes clear.

Transition to Next Chapter

Now that you understand how diagnosis is made, the next step is treatment, starting with non-surgical options.

CHAPTER 16: Managing Without Surgery – What Helps, What Does Not, and What to Expect

The Question Everyone Wants Answered

Once a diagnosis is made, most patients ask:

"Can I avoid surgery?"

It is a very natural concern. Surgery is not something people choose easily.

The honest answer is:

In some situations, yes. In many cases, only for a limited time.

Non-surgical treatment can help, especially in early or mild cases. But it is important to understand clearly where it works and where it does not.

When Non-Surgical Management Is Reasonable

There are situations where surgery is not immediately necessary.

These include:

Gallstones without symptoms

Mild and infrequent symptoms

Medical reasons to delay surgery

Patient preference after understanding risks

In these cases, careful observation and management can be appropriate.

Managing Pain During an Episode

During a gallbladder attack, the first goal is relief.

This may include:

Pain-relieving medications

Rest

Avoiding food during the episode

Pain usually improves as the temporary blockage resolves.

However, it is important to remember:

Pain relief treats symptoms, not the underlying cause.

Hydration and Supportive Care

In more significant episodes:

Adequate hydration is important

Light or no food may be needed temporarily

In hospital settings, intravenous fluids may be given if symptoms are more severe.

Diet – Helpful but Not a Cure

Diet plays an important role but is often misunderstood.

A low-fat diet can:

Reduce gallbladder stimulation

Decrease frequency of attacks

Patients are often advised to avoid:

Fried foods

Greasy meals

Large heavy portions

However, diet does not remove existing gallstones.

It helps control symptoms, not eliminate the problem.

Medications to Dissolve Stones

Certain medications can dissolve specific types of gallstones.

However:

They work only in selected cases

They require long-term use

Stones may return

Because of these limitations, they are not commonly used.

Guidance from the National Institute of Diabetes and Digestive and Kidney Diseases supports their limited role.

Antibiotics – When They Are Needed

Antibiotics are not used for simple gallstone pain.

They are used when:

Infection is present

Conditions like cholecystitis or cholangitis occur

Unnecessary use does not help and may cause side effects.

Watchful Waiting – A Valid Approach

For patients with silent gallstones, watchful waiting is often recommended.

This means:

No immediate treatment

Monitoring for symptoms

Seeking care if symptoms develop

Many people live without ever needing treatment.

When Non-Surgical Treatment Is Not Enough

There are clear situations where conservative management is not sufficient.

These include:

Recurrent attacks

Persistent symptoms

Complications such as inflammation or duct stones

In these cases, delaying definitive treatment may increase risk.

A Common Mistake to Avoid

A frequent mistake is relying only on temporary relief.

Patients may:

Take medications

Modify diet briefly

Ignore recurring symptoms

This often delays proper treatment.

A Practical Way to Think About It

A simple approach is:

No symptoms → observe

Mild symptoms → manage and monitor

Recurrent symptoms → consider definitive treatment

Balancing Expectations

It is important to be realistic.

Non-surgical treatment:

Can reduce symptoms

Can delay surgery

Usually cannot prevent recurrence

Your Role in Decision-Making

You play an important role.

Consider:

Frequency of symptoms

Severity

Impact on daily life

Discuss these openly with your doctor.

A Thought from My Practice

I often tell my patients:

It is not about avoiding surgery at all costs. It is about choosing the right treatment at the right time.

Chapter Summary

Non-surgical management can help in selected patients, especially those with mild or no symptoms. However, it does not remove gallstones. Recurrent or severe symptoms usually require definitive treatment.

Action Plan

If symptoms are mild, follow dietary advice and monitor patterns. If symptoms recur, do not rely only on temporary relief. Discuss long-term options.

Transition to Next Chapter

Now that you understand non-surgical options, the next step is to look at the most effective and definitive treatment, surgery.

CHAPTER 17: Gallbladder Surgery – Understanding the Definitive Treatment

When Treatment Becomes Clear

By now, a pattern should be clear.

Gallstones may remain silent for years. But once they begin to cause repeated symptoms, the problem usually returns.

At that stage, the question is no longer what is happening. It becomes what is the most reliable way to fix it.

For most symptomatic patients, the answer is gallbladder removal, also called cholecystectomy.

Why Removing the Gallbladder Works

This is an important concept.

The gallbladder is the place where:

Stones form

Bile is stored

Blockage occurs

When the gallbladder is removed:

Stones cannot form there again

The source of repeated attacks is removed

This is why surgery is considered a definitive treatment.

Guidance from the National Institute of Diabetes and Digestive and Kidney Diseases supports this approach.

When Is Surgery Recommended

Surgery is not needed for everyone.

It is usually recommended when:

There are repeated attacks

Symptoms affect daily life

Complications have developed

Stones are present in the bile duct

Symptoms persist despite treatment

The decision is based on symptoms, not just the presence of stones.

Types of Gallbladder Surgery

There are two main approaches.

Laparoscopic Cholecystectomy

This is the most common method.

It involves:

Small incisions

A camera and specialized instruments

Removal of the gallbladder with minimal disruption

Benefits include:

Less pain

Faster recovery

Short hospital stay

Most patients undergo this procedure.

Open Cholecystectomy

This is a traditional method.

It involves:

A larger incision

Direct access to the gallbladder

It may be needed when:

There are complications

Anatomy is unclear

Laparoscopic surgery is not possible

Recovery is longer.

What Happens During Surgery

The procedure is done under anesthesia.

In simple terms:

The gallbladder is identified

It is carefully separated

It is removed safely

Nearby structures are checked

The procedure usually takes one to two hours.

Is Gallbladder Surgery Safe

This is a common concern.

Gallbladder surgery is one of the most commonly performed operations worldwide.

In experienced hands:

It is generally safe

Serious complications are uncommon

Possible Risks

Although uncommon, risks may include:

Bleeding

Infection

Injury to nearby structures

Leakage of bile

Your surgeon will explain these clearly.

Gallbladder Surgery

Cholecystectomy

(removal of the gallbladder)

Laparoscopic Surgery

Open Surgery

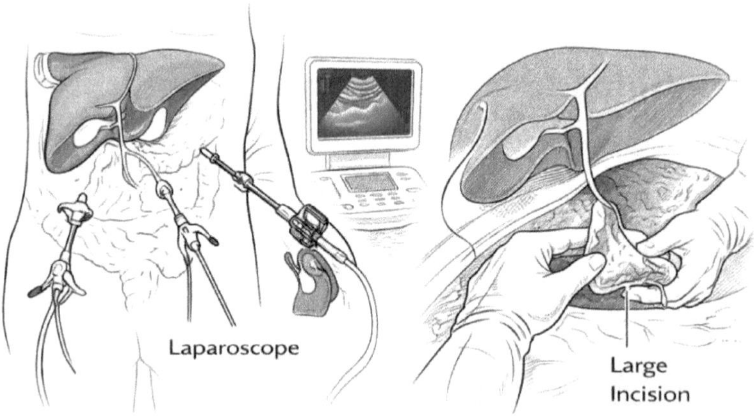

Small Incisions

Dector cheeks
for tenderness |

Usce sound waves to create images of the gallbladder and bile ducts.

The gallbladder is not necessary for digestion, and its removal usually resolves symptoms of gallbladder

Preparing for Surgery

Preparation is straightforward.

You may be advised to:

Avoid food for several hours before surgery

Adjust certain medications

Complete basic tests

Hospital Stay and Recovery

For laparoscopic surgery:

Many patients go home the same day or next day

Early movement is encouraged

Most patients:

Resume light activities within a few days

Return to work within one to two weeks

Open surgery requires longer recovery.

Life Without a Gallbladder

Many patients worry about this.

The reassuring truth is:

The liver continues to produce bile

Digestion continues normally

Some temporary changes may occur but usually improve.

Why Surgery Prevents Recurrence

Once the gallbladder is removed:

The environment for stone formation is gone

Recurrent attacks are prevented

Making the Decision

The decision should be:

Thoughtful

Based on symptoms and risk

Made in consultation with your doctor

There is no need to rush, but also no need to delay unnecessarily.

A Thought from My Practice

I often tell my patients:

If the gallbladder is causing repeated problems, removing it removes the problem.

Chapter Summary

Gallbladder surgery is the most effective treatment for symptomatic gallstones. Laparoscopic surgery is commonly used and allows faster recovery. Removing the gallbladder prevents recurrence.

Action Plan

If surgery is recommended, understand the reasons clearly. Ask questions and prepare well. Follow instructions carefully.

Transition to Next Chapter

Now that you understand surgery, the next step is to know what happens after it and how life adjusts.

CHAPTER 18: Life After Gallbladder Removal – What Really Changes

A Natural Concern

By this stage, many patients ask:

"Will I be normal after my gallbladder is removed?"

It is a very reasonable concern.

The reassuring answer is:

Yes, in most cases, life returns to normal.

There may be a short period of adjustment, but the body adapts well.

What Changes Inside the Body

Before surgery:

The liver produces bile

The gallbladder stores and releases it during meals

After surgery:

The liver continues to produce bile

There is no storage

Bile flows continuously into the intestine

Although this seems like a big change, the body adjusts effectively.

The First Few Days – Early Recovery

In the first few days, it is normal to experience:

Mild pain at the incision sites

Tiredness

Reduced appetite

Some bloating

These symptoms improve steadily.

The First Few Weeks – Adjustment Phase

As recovery continues, the digestive system adapts.

During this time, you may notice:

Sensitivity to heavy meals

Occasional loose stools

A feeling of fullness

These changes are usually temporary.

Understanding Post-Surgery Diarrhea

A small number of patients experience loose stools.

This happens because:

Bile enters the intestine continuously

It may stimulate bowel movement

Important points:

It is usually mild

It improves over time

It can be managed with diet

Diet After Surgery – A Practical Approach

In the early phase:

Start with light, simple foods

Eat small, frequent meals

Gradually:

Return to normal foods

Reintroduce fats slowly

Avoid heavy, greasy meals initially.

Long-Term Eating – No Extreme Restrictions

After recovery:

No strict diet is required

Most foods can be eaten in moderation

Focus on:

Balanced meals

Reasonable portions

Consistency

Returning to Normal Activities

Recovery after laparoscopic surgery is usually quick.

Most patients:

Start walking within a day

Resume light activity within a few days

Return to work within one to two weeks

Strenuous activity should be avoided initially.

When to Seek Medical Advice

Contact your doctor if you notice:

Increasing pain

Fever

Redness or discharge from the wound

Persistent vomiting

Severe or prolonged diarrhea

Long-Term Outlook

The long-term outlook is excellent.

Most patients:

Experience relief from symptoms

Eat normally

Live active lives

Emotional Adjustment

It is normal to feel some anxiety after surgery.

Remember:

Recovery happens step by step

The body adapts well

Confidence returns quickly

A Simple Way to Understand It

The gallbladder is helpful, but not essential.

A Thought from My Practice

Patients who understand what to expect after surgery recover with more confidence and less anxiety.

Chapter Summary

After gallbladder removal, bile flows continuously instead of being stored. Most patients recover quickly and return to normal life. Temporary digestive changes may occur but improve over time.

Action Plan

Follow a light diet initially. Gradually return to normal eating. Stay active but avoid strain early. Seek advice if symptoms persist.

Transition to Next Chapter

Now that you understand life after surgery, the next step is to focus on long-term habits that support digestive health.

CHAPTER 19: Diet, Weight, and Lifestyle – Building Long-Term Digestive Health

From Treatment to Everyday Living

By now, you have a clear understanding of gallbladder disease and its treatment.

This chapter shifts the focus to daily life. It is about simple habits that support digestion and reduce future risk.

In my experience, patients who adopt steady, realistic habits do far better than those who try strict plans briefly and then abandon them.

A Balanced Diet – Not a Perfect Diet

You do not need a perfect diet. You need a balanced one.

A practical approach includes:

Moderate intake of fats

Plenty of fruits and vegetables

Whole grains

Lean sources of protein

This is not about restriction. It is about consistency.

Understanding Fat Intake

Fat plays an important role in gallbladder function.

Too much fat:

Can trigger strong gallbladder contraction

May cause symptoms

Too little fat for long periods:

May reduce gallbladder emptying

May contribute to stone formation

The goal is balance.

Better choices include:

Olive oil

Nuts in moderation

Fish

Limit:

Fried foods

Processed meals

Large, heavy portions

Meal Timing – A Simple but Powerful Habit

How you eat matters.

Helpful habits include:

Eating at regular times

Avoiding long gaps between meals

Not skipping meals frequently

Regular eating supports better bile flow.

Weight Management – A Key Factor

Body weight is an important factor.

Important points:

Excess weight increases cholesterol in bile

Rapid weight loss also increases risk

The best approach is:

Gradual, steady weight control

Avoiding crash diets

Guidance from the National Institute of Diabetes and Digestive and Kidney Diseases supports this.

Physical Activity – Simple and Effective

Regular activity helps:

Maintain weight

Improve digestion

Support overall health

Simple options include:

Walking

Light exercise

Staying active during the day

Consistency is more important than intensity.

Hydration – Often Overlooked

Adequate water intake supports:

Digestion

Metabolism

Overall health

Make hydration a regular habit.

Avoiding Common Mistakes

Common mistakes include:

Following extreme diets

Eliminating fats completely

Ignoring symptoms

Relying on unproven remedies

A balanced, evidence-based approach works best.

Gallbladder Health

Diet, Weight, and Lifestyle Changes

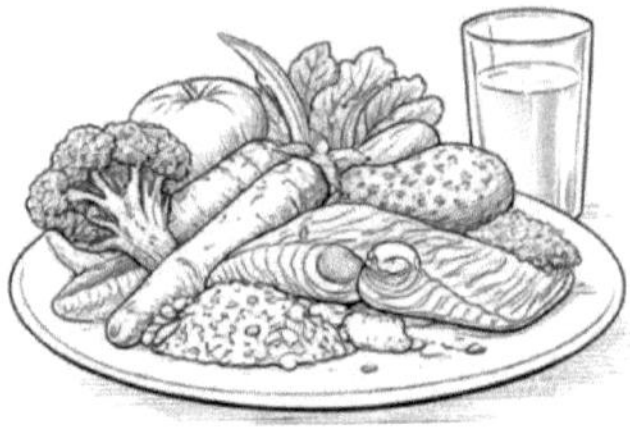

Eat a Healthy Diet

Choose foods rich in fiber, low in saturated fats, and avoid fried or greasy foods.

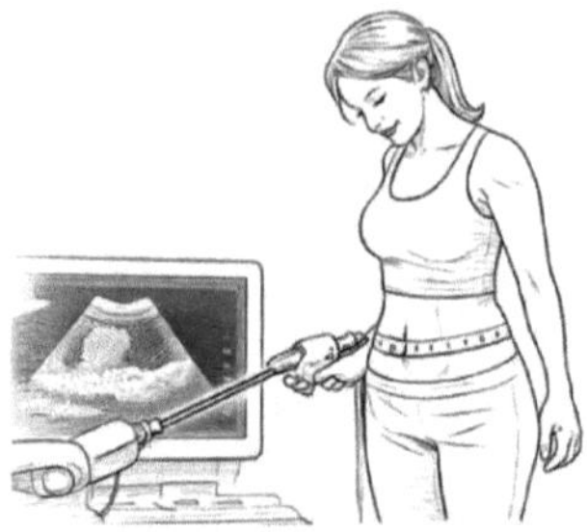

Maintain a Healthy Weight

Maintain a healthy weight to reduce the risk of gallstones.

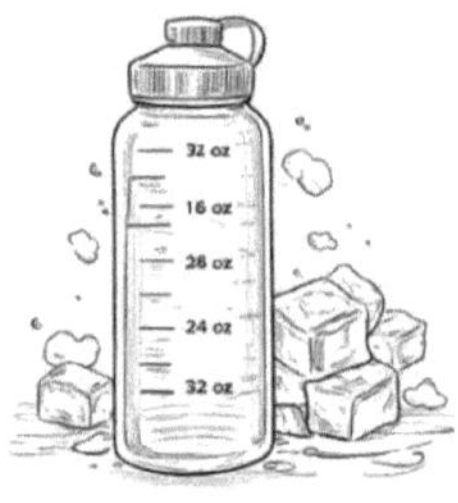

Stay Hydrated

Drink plenty of water throughout the day to help bile flow and prevent gallstones

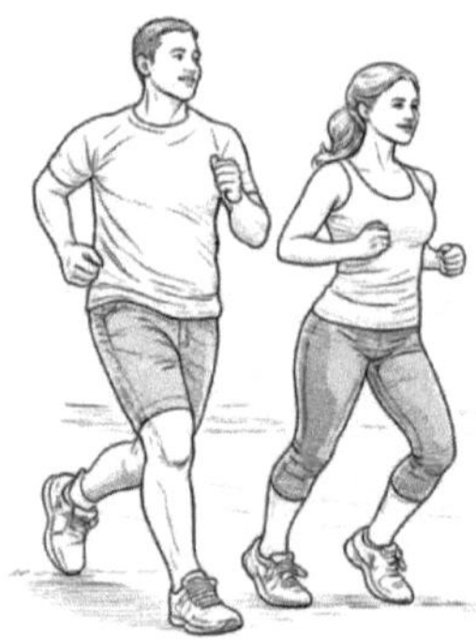

Exercise Regularly

Get regular physical activity to maintain weight and support overall digestive health.

After Surgery – Why Lifestyle Still Matters

Even after gallbladder removal:

Healthy habits remain important

They:

Support digestion

Prevent other metabolic problems

Improve overall well-being

Can Gallstones Be Prevented Completely

Complete prevention is not always possible.

However, risk can be reduced by:

Maintaining a healthy weight

Eating balanced meals

Staying active

Avoiding rapid weight loss

Building a Sustainable Routine

A simple routine includes:

Regular meals

Moderate portions

Daily activity

Adequate hydration

These habits are effective and sustainable.

A Practical Perspective

You do not need perfection. You need consistency.

Small, steady habits make a lasting difference.

A Thought from My Practice

Patients who adopt simple lifestyle changes often feel better overall, not just in digestion but in energy and well-being.

Chapter Summary

Diet, weight, and lifestyle play a central role in managing and preventing gallbladder disease. Balanced eating, steady weight control, and regular activity are key.

Action Plan

Adopt a balanced diet. Maintain a healthy weight gradually. Stay active. Avoid extreme dietary patterns. Focus on habits you can sustain.

Transition to Next Chapter

Now that you understand long-term lifestyle measures, the next step is to look at special situations where care needs to be individualized.

CHAPTER 20: Special Situations and High-Risk Groups – When Care Needs to Be Individualized

Why One Approach Does Not Fit Everyone

By now, you have a strong understanding of gallbladder disease.

But in real-life practice, no two patients are exactly alike.

Age, medical conditions, pregnancy, and weight changes can all influence symptoms, risks, and treatment decisions.

One important principle guides good care:

Treatment should always be individualized.

Older Adults – Subtle Symptoms, Higher Risk

Gallstones are more common with increasing age.

In older adults:

Symptoms may be less obvious

Pain may be mild or atypical

Weakness may be more noticeable than pain

At the same time:

Complications can develop more quickly

Recovery may take longer

Careful evaluation is essential.

Patients with Diabetes – A Need for Extra Care

Diabetes affects how the body responds to illness.

In these patients:

Symptoms may be less pronounced

Infections may develop more easily

Complications may progress faster

Doctors often take a more cautious approach to avoid serious outcomes.

Pregnancy – A Unique Situation

Pregnancy affects the gallbladder due to hormonal changes.

These changes:

Slow gallbladder emptying

Increase cholesterol in bile

This raises the risk of gallstones.

Most cases are managed conservatively.

However:

Severe symptoms may require intervention

Surgery, when necessary, can be performed safely

Rapid Weight Loss and Bariatric Surgery

Rapid weight loss is an important risk factor.

It:

Increases cholesterol release into bile

Reduces gallbladder activity

This may occur:

With crash diets

After bariatric surgery

Preventive strategies may be considered in selected patients.

Patients with Liver Disease

The liver produces bile, so liver disease can affect gallbladder function.

In these patients:

Bile composition may change

Pigment stones may form

Treatment decisions require careful consideration

Critically Ill Patients – Acalculous Cholecystitis

In severely ill patients, gallbladder inflammation may occur without stones.

This is called acalculous cholecystitis.

It is associated with:

Severe illness

Reduced blood flow

Prolonged hospitalization

Early recognition is important.

Gallbladder Disease in Children

Although less common, gallbladder disease can occur in children.

Possible causes include:

Genetic factors

Blood disorders

Obesity

Symptoms are similar but require careful evaluation.

Medications and Hormonal Factors

Certain medications may increase risk.

Examples include:

Hormonal therapies

Some cholesterol-related medications

Awareness is helpful, but medications should not be stopped without medical advice.

Why Individualized Care Matters

Every patient's situation is different.

Treatment decisions depend on:

Age

Overall health

Severity of symptoms

Presence of complications

Personal preferences

There is no single plan for everyone.

A Practical Way to Understand It

Different situations require different approaches.

For example:

A young healthy person may recover quickly from surgery

An older patient may need a more cautious plan

Pregnancy requires careful timing

Diabetes requires closer monitoring

A Thought from My Practice

Patients who understand their individual risks are more confident and make better decisions.

Chapter Summary

Gallbladder disease behaves differently in special situations such as older age, diabetes, pregnancy, rapid weight loss, and liver disease. These require individualized care.

Action Plan

Inform your doctor about all medical conditions and medications. Understand how your situation affects your care. Follow medical advice carefully.

Transition to Next Chapter

Now that we have discussed special situations, the next step is to address common questions that patients frequently ask.

CHAPTER 21: Common Questions – Simple, Clear, and Honest Answers

Why This Chapter Matters

Even after understanding symptoms, diagnosis, and treatment, most patients still have questions.

These questions are important. They often come from personal experiences, conversations with others, or information found online.

Some are based on facts. Others are based on misunderstandings.

Clear answers replace uncertainty with confidence.

Do All Gallstones Need Surgery

No.

If gallstones:

Are not causing symptoms

Are found incidentally

then they often do not require immediate treatment.

However, once symptoms begin and especially if they recur, surgery becomes the most effective long-term solution.

Can Gallstones Go Away on Their Own

In most cases, no.

Gallstones usually remain unless treated.

Some medications may dissolve certain stones, but:

They work only in selected cases

They take time

Stones may return

Can Diet Cure Gallstones

Diet helps manage symptoms, but it does not cure gallstones.

A healthy diet can:

Reduce frequency of attacks

Improve digestion

But it does not remove existing stones.

Is Gallbladder Surgery Safe

Yes, in most cases.

Laparoscopic gallbladder surgery is widely performed and generally safe.

As with any surgery:

There are risks

But serious complications are uncommon

Will I Be Able to Eat Normally After Surgery

This is a very common concern.

Most people:

Return to a normal diet

Eat a wide variety of foods

Do not require long-term restrictions

Some may need a short adjustment period.

Can Gallstones Come Back After Surgery

Once the gallbladder is removed:

Stones do not form in it again

In rare cases, stones may form in the bile ducts.

Can Gallbladder Pain Be Mistaken for Gas or Acidity

Yes, very often.

Gallbladder pain can resemble:

Gas

Indigestion

Acid reflux

However:

It is usually more intense

It follows a pattern

It is often related to meals

What Happens If I Ignore My Symptoms

Ignoring symptoms may lead to:

Repeated attacks

Increasing severity

Complications such as infection or pancreatitis

Early care usually leads to better outcomes.

Do Natural Remedies Help

Many patients ask about natural or herbal treatments.

Some may support digestion, but:

There is no strong evidence they remove gallstones

Relying only on them may delay proper treatment

How Do I Decide About Surgery

This is a personal decision.

Consider:

Frequency of symptoms

Severity

Impact on daily life

Risk of complications

Discuss these with your doctor.

What Should I Ask My Doctor

Helpful questions include:

What is causing my symptoms

Do I need surgery now

What are my options

What are the risks and benefits

A Practical Perspective

Unanswered questions create unnecessary anxiety. Clear answers bring confidence.

A Thought from My Practice

Patients who ask questions and understand their condition make better decisions and feel more comfortable with their care.

Chapter Summary

Many common concerns about gallbladder disease can be answered clearly. Not all gallstones need surgery, but symptomatic ones usually do. Diet helps but does not cure the condition.

Action Plan

Write down your questions before visits. Seek clear answers. Avoid relying on unverified information. Make informed decisions.

Transition to Next Chapter

In the final chapter, we will bring everything together, clear common myths, and leave you with a confident approach to your health.

CHAPTER 22: Myths, Facts, and Final Thoughts – A Calm, Confident Way Forward

Clearing the Last Layer of Confusion

As we reach the end of this book, there is one final step that matters.

Even after understanding the science, many patients carry lingering beliefs. These may come from friends, online sources, or past experiences.

Some are harmless. Others can influence decisions in the wrong direction.

So let us take a moment to clear them calmly and clearly.

Myth 1: All Gallstones Must Be Removed Immediately

Fact:

Many gallstones are silent.

If you have no symptoms:

Observation is often enough

But once symptoms begin:

Treatment becomes relevant

Balanced decisions are always better than rushed ones.

Myth 2: Surgery Should Always Be Avoided

Fact:

Avoiding surgery is not always the safest choice.

When symptoms are repeated:

The problem is ongoing

The risk of complications increases

In such cases, surgery becomes a solution, not something to fear.

Myth 3: Life Will Not Be Normal After Gallbladder Removal

Fact:

Most people return to normal life.

The body adapts:

The liver continues to produce bile

Digestion continues

Temporary changes may occur, but long-term issues are uncommon.

Myth 4: Only Fatty Food Causes Gallstones

Fact:

Diet is only one part of the picture.

Other factors include:

Body weight

Hormones

Genetics

Metabolism

Blaming diet alone oversimplifies the condition.

Myth 5: Natural Remedies Can Cure Gallstones

Fact:

There is no strong scientific evidence that natural remedies can remove gallstones.

Some may support digestion, but they do not eliminate stones.

Reliable guidance from the National Institute of Diabetes and Digestive and Kidney Diseases supports evidence-based treatment.

Myth 6: Gallbladder Disease Is Always Mild

Fact:

While many cases are mild, some can become serious.

Complications may include:

Infection

Bile duct blockage

Pancreatitis

Early recognition is important.

Myth 7: Pain Will Eventually Go Away Permanently

Fact:

Pain may settle temporarily, but it often returns.

Repeated episodes usually indicate ongoing disease.

Looking Back – What You Have Learned

Let us pause and reflect.

You now understand:

How the gallbladder works

How gallstones form

Why symptoms occur

How diagnosis is made

When treatment is needed

What surgery involves

What to expect after treatment

How lifestyle affects long-term health

This is not just information. It is clarity.

What Truly Matters Going Forward

A few simple principles make a real difference:

Pay attention to your body

Recognize patterns

Seek medical advice when needed

Avoid panic and avoid neglect

Make decisions based on clear information

A Calm and Practical Approach

You do not need to worry about every symptom.

But you should not ignore repeated ones.

Stay aware. Stay balanced. Act when needed.

Your Role in Your Own Health

You can take charge by:

Understanding your condition

Asking the right questions

Following practical advice

Staying consistent with healthy habits

A Final Thought from My Practice

After many years of caring for patients, one pattern stands out.

Patients who:

Understand their condition

Act at the right time

Follow simple, steady habits

almost always do well.

Gallbladder disease, in most cases, is treatable and manageable.

Chapter Summary

Many common beliefs about gallbladder disease are incorrect. Most gallstones are silent, surgery is safe when needed, and life after treatment is usually normal. Awareness and timely action lead to the best outcomes.

Final Action Plan

Stay aware of symptoms

Seek timely medical advice

Make informed decisions

Maintain healthy habits

Avoid misinformation

Closing Note

Good health is not only about treatment.

It is about understanding, awareness, and timely action.

You now have that understanding.

Move forward with clarity, confidence, and peace of mind.

APPENDIX A: A Simple Guide to the Gallbladder and Bile System

Why This Matters

In my experience, once patients can visualize what is happening inside their body, everything becomes easier to understand.

Pain feels less confusing. Test results make more sense. Decisions feel more logical.

You do not need complex anatomy. A simple picture is enough.

The Gallbladder – A Small but Important Organ

The gallbladder is a small, pear-shaped organ located under the liver on the right side of the abdomen.

Its role is to:

Store bile

Concentrate bile

Release bile during meals

Think of it as a storage pouch that helps digestion.

The Liver – The Source of Bile

The liver produces bile continuously.

Bile contains:

Bile salts for fat digestion

Cholesterol

Bilirubin

Water and other substances

The gallbladder does not produce bile. It only stores and releases it.

The Bile Ducts – The Pathway

Bile flows through a system of ducts.

This includes:

Small ducts within the liver

Hepatic ducts

Cystic duct connecting the gallbladder

Common bile duct leading to the intestine

This pathway is essential for digestion.

How the System Works

A simple sequence:

The liver produces bile

The gallbladder stores it

During meals, the gallbladder contracts

Bile flows into the intestine

Fat is digested

What Happens When There Is a Problem

Problems occur when:

Stones form

Ducts are blocked

The gallbladder does not empty properly

This leads to:

Pain

Inflammation

Infection

The Link with the Pancreas

The bile duct joins the pancreatic duct before entering the intestine.

Because of this:

A stone can affect both systems

This explains gallstone pancreatitis

Appendix Summary

Liver makes bile

Gallbladder stores bile

Ducts carry bile

Blockage causes symptoms

Practical Takeaway

Think of the flow:

Liver → Gallbladder → Ducts → Intestine

This simple model helps you understand the entire condition.

APPENDIX B: Understanding Your Test Reports – Blood Tests and Imaging

Why This Matters

Medical reports can look complex.

Once you understand what doctors are looking for, they become much easier to interpret.

What Doctors Are Trying to Find

Doctors are looking for:

Gallstones

Inflammation

Blockage

Involvement of other organs

Blood Tests – What They Show

Common tests include:

Liver function tests:

Bilirubin → suggests blockage

AST/ALT → liver stress

ALP → bile duct obstruction

CBC:

High white blood cells → infection

Pancreatic enzymes:

Elevated levels → pancreatitis

Imaging Tests

Ultrasound:

First test

Detects stones and inflammation

HIDA scan:

Assesses function

CT scan:

Detects complications

MRCP:

Visualizes bile ducts

ERCP:

Diagnoses and treats duct stones

Common Terms in Reports

Gallstones → stones present

Sludge → thick bile

Wall thickening → inflammation

Dilated duct → blockage

Practical Takeaway

Do not panic when reading reports.

Always interpret them in discussion with your doctor.

APPENDIX C: Preparing for Gallbladder Surgery – A Practical Checklist

Why Preparation Matters

Patients who prepare well feel calmer and recover faster.

Questions to Ask

Why is surgery needed

Can it wait

What type of surgery will be done

What are the risks

What is recovery like

Before Surgery

Follow fasting instructions

Review medications

Arrange help at home

Plan rest after surgery

After Surgery Planning

Start with a light diet

Gradually return to activity

Attend follow-up visits

Practical Takeaway

Preparation reduces anxiety and improves recovery.

APPENDIX D: Recovery After Surgery – A Simple Guide

Early Recovery

Rest

Light diet

Pain control

First Week

Gentle walking

Gradual increase in activity

Monitor wound

Warning Signs

Seek medical advice if:

Fever

Increasing pain

Wound infection

Persistent vomiting

Practical Takeaway

Recovery is usually smooth when simple steps are followed.

APPENDIX E: Symptom Tracker and Red Flag Guide

What to Track

Time of symptoms

Pain location

Relation to meals

Duration

Associated symptoms

When to Seek Help

Mild symptoms:

Monitor at home

Persistent symptoms:

Contact your doctor

Severe symptoms:

Seek emergency care

A Simple Rule

Mild → Monitor

Persistent → Call

Severe → Emergency

Practical Takeaway

Tracking symptoms helps early diagnosis and better care.

Thank You and Please Review the Book

Thank you for taking the time to read this book. I sincerely hope it has helped you understand your health a little more clearly and has given you practical, everyday steps you can follow with confidence. If you found this book helpful, **I would truly appreciate it if you could leave a brief and honest review.** Even a few lines sharing your experience can make a meaningful difference. Your feedback helps other readers find reliable, trustworthy health information and supports them in making better decisions for themselves and their families.

Warm regards,

Dr Prabhat Das

Continue your Healthcare Journey

Good health is a journey, not a single step. It is not achieved in one day or with one book. That is why I created the "Better Health with Dr Das" series, with each book addressing a different common condition. If you would like easy, practical guidance on other everyday health concerns, you may wish to explore the rest of books in this series.

Books in this series:

Better Health starts Here: A Doctor's Guide to Staying Healthy After 40

A Doctor's Easy Guide to Understanding & Managing OBESITY

Doctor, What DIET Is Best for Me?

Doctor, Why Can't I Lose Weight? A Doctor's Guide to safe & Sustainable Weight Loss)

A Doctor's Easy Guide to GLP-1 for Obesity

A Doctor's Easy Guide to Understanding & Managing HIGH BLOOD PRESSURE

A Doctor's Guide to Living Well With DIABETES

A Doctor's Guide to Understanding & Managing THYROID DISEASES

A Doctor's Guide to Understanding & Managing HIGH CHOLESTEROL

A Doctor's Practical Guide to HEART HEALTH After 40: How to Protect Your Heart & Live Longer

A Doctor's Guide to Healing & Reversing FATTY LIVER DISEASE: Simple, Natural & Science-Based Steps to Reduce Liver Fat and Prevent Complications

Control Your ACID REFLUX, HEARTBURN & GERD: A Doctor's Practical Guide that Works

Live Comfortably with IRRITABLE BOWEL SYNDROME: A Doctor's Practical Guide to Understanding & Managing IBS

A Doctor's Practical Guide to Understanding & Managing GALLBLADDER STONES & OTHER PROBLEMS

Take Control of COPD: A Doctor's Practical Guide to Better Breathing

Living Better Life with ASTHMA: A Doctor's Practical Guide to Asthma Control

SLEEP APNEA & SNORING: A Doctor's Practical Guide to Better Sleep & Better Health

KIDNEY STONES: A Doctor's Practical Guide to Prevention & Care

Protect Your KIDNEYS: A Doctor's Practical Guide to Kidney Health & Prevention

PROSTATE HEALTH After 40: A Doctor's Practical Guide to Early Detection & Care

ARTHRITIS: A Doctor's Practical Guide to Pain Control & Mobility

A Doctor's Practical Guide to Fixing BACK PAIN Step by Step

A Doctor's Practical Guide to Understanding & Managing GOUT & URIC ACID and Preventing Complications

HEALTHY SKIN & COMMON SKIN PROBLEMS: A Doctor's Practical Guide to Skin Care

DEMENTIA & MEMORY LOSS: A Doctor's Practical Guide to Prevention & Management

Doctor, Why Am I TIRED All The Time? Fixing Fatigue & Getting Your Energy Back

9 781971 672335

Printed by Libri Plureos GmbH in Hamburg, Germany